Keeping Work Simple

500 Tips, Rules, and Tools

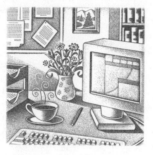

Don Aslett
and
Carol Cartaino

A Storey Publishing Book

STOREY

Storey Communications, Inc.
Schoolhouse Road
Pownal, Vermont 05261

*The mission of Storey Communications is to serve our
customers by publishing practical information that
encourages personal independence in harmony with
the environment.*

Edited by William Overstreet and Gwen Steege
Cover design by Meredith Maker
Cover illustration by Paul Hoffman
Text design by Greg Imhoff and Susan Bernier
Production by Erin Lincourt
Indexed by Northwind Editorial Services

Printed in the United States by Vicks Lithograph
10 9 8 7 6 5 4 3 2 1

Library of Congress Cataloging-in-Publication Data

Aslett, Don, 1935–
        Keeping work simple / Don Aslett and Carol Cartaino.
             p.   cm.
        Includes index.
        ISBN 0-88266-996-6 (pbk. : alk. paper)
        1. Time management.   2. Self-management (Psychology)
3. Stress (Psychology)   4. Job stress.   I. Cartaino, Carol, 1944– .
II. Title.
    BF637.T5A85   1997
    640—dc21   97-13736
                                                         CIP

Contents

Acknowledgments

For helping to make this book possible, we would like to thank:

Oscar Collier, who provided moral support, wisdom from his own office experience, and a sounding board when needed.

Martha Jacob and Jenny Behymer, who helped gather nuggets of know-how from the wide world of the office.

Tobi Haynes, Michael Patton Hoover, Judi Mills, and Susan Waddell, who shared their knowledge at length.

Grandma Ann Cartaino, who made child care simple while Mother was "Making Work Simple."

And the other many others who cheerfully contributed their time and expertise, including:

Marylyn Alexander, Ellen Cartaino, Linda Chaney, Shirley Creek, Jim Doles, Leon King, Marcia Kirk, Charles C. Krainz, Jr., Cathy Judge, Barbara McAnanich, Pauline Marsh, Rose Fisher Merkowitz, Ed Rach, Karen Reno, Angela and Peter Seidel, Senter Office Supply, Barbara Shoemaker, Ernest Smalley, Hollis Stevenson, Marilyn M. Stewart, Dave Stoddard, Richard Van Zant, Kevin Watts, and Darlene Yuellig.

A Note to the Reader

After collaboration on twenty-five books since 1980, it was time to author one together. Carol Cartaino was editor-in-chief for a well-known publisher when my first amateur, self-published book (*Is There Life After Housework?*) passed through her office. She recognized it as a diamond in the rough, worked it over, and it went on to be a million seller. Then she suggested I write another book, in a question-and-answer format, and masterfully edited it (*Do I Dust or Vacuum First?*) into a book that sold a half million more. Twenty-three others of my books (Cartainoized) followed, and thanks to her genius and application, they have succeeded, too.

Now an independent freelance editor and writer/collaborator, she contributes to all of my books, brochures, and corporate printed material. Never accepting anything but the best, she toils until midnight with marker pens and computer, to make manuscripts come alive in every line and paragraph.

So when a request came from another premier publisher for a book about simplifying work, a subject we both loved and had considerable credibility in, we decided to partner No. #26, this present volume. True to all the other books we've worked on, first she pulled everything I had to say about the subject out of me, and boiled down and polished the free-flowing drafts that resulted. Then she added more ideas, examples, stories, and nuts and bolts of her own. She also tapped her gallery of the best office workers she knew, from secretaries to office-supply stores, postmasters to production chiefs. Then she sifted, blended, and mixed, and *WE* have a book, a good one, with lots of fresh, new, and workable advice for making work simple!

Don Aslett

Introduction

An idea persists in some quarters that once you work your way to an office position, you've reached an easy job. Some people still assume that those assembly line laborers or field hands worked and studied hard enough to finally merit an "office" position, so now they have it made. But after looking through the office window from both sides now for more than forty years, I'd give office work a solid three-to-one vote for being the tougher taskmaster.

I grew up working in the fields and barns of a large ranch and in sundry construction trades — long, backbreaking hours in 110-degree heat and 45-degree-below-zero cold, wrestling two thousand pound bulls, herding and hauling hundreds of hogs, and running harvesters and other machinery in dust and noise that would make a sandstorm look soothing. I was a licensed painter, mason, janitor, builder before I was old enough to vote. Twelve-hour work days were short ones to me, and sixteen-to-eighteen hour ones not unheard of. Yet I only felt tired, never weary, at the end of the day. I worked outside, with others, and looked forward eagerly to each new day — muscle work is relaxing, rewarding, restoring.

Then I went to college, one theme was pounded into us: "Grow smart so you don't have to do grunt work." We all looked forward to the day when we could put on a suit, pick up a briefcase, and take our place at the desk of authority. Then came the surprise. The local high school needed an English and speech teacher and coach. The combination of my education and past experience made me well qualified. I thought, HA! the promise fulfilled, an office... inside, intellectual work at last! I accepted. I only had to be there from 8:30 A.M. to 3:30 P.M. and had one free period and lunchtime off — the lightest workday imaginable!

Two weeks later, as I was lying on the couch one evening at 6:00 P.M., too exhausted to get up and eat supper, my wife thought for sure I had developed hepatitis. When I came home from those few hours of white-collar work I was tense, spent, beaten down, exhausted. This was without question the hardest work I'd ever done. Mental work, emotional work, office work. They take their toll.

In the office we often don't have a stern overseer standing over us. Instead, we fight the much harder battle of self-discipline. We're around others all the time but have to carefully monitor what we say and do — no blowing off steam and too little fraternity. We work in confined spaces and often don't see the sun except on the way to and from work. We dress fancy, keep fit on our own time, and endure all kinds of mental hassles and pressures.

Recently, I observed the CEO of my cleaning company during a week of ordinary days at the office. The phone constantly brought bad news, often forcing him to make tough decisions. Visitors, salespeople, auditors, and accountants formed lines to see him. Mail came in by the cartload. Scouts, Rotary, and community causes were waiting. Lawyers petitioned him about minority, equality, and arbitration problems. And then there were all those staff meetings and conferences. The job literally had no beginning or end, just constant demands for his time and attention. A week later I heard his eighteen-year-old daughter describing her dad's job. "Oh," she said, "he has this big office and sits in a big soft chair behind a desk answering the phone."

Office work, for any who do it now or will do it someday, is not time off. Negotiating and directing the traffic in an office, whether at home or downtown, adds up to big-time brutality, which makes it a worthy target for taming. And it can be done! How? *By simplifying.* That's what this book is meant to do — to help you find ways to make office work easier, simpler, and even fun!

You won't find in this book a conscientious compilation of what other writers and sources have to say. The ideas and suggestions in here all come from real life, from people who have put in their time on the ramparts — in the cubicles, at the desk, on the phone, and at the keyboard.

You don't have to agree with everything in here to benefit. Even a half-dozen new insights or ideas out of this whole book can reward you a thousand times over, if they simplify and improve your life at the office!

Don Aslett

Cleaning Your Slate

In this chapter . . .

- *Why Clean Counts*
- *Doing Things Now*
- *Clearing That Backlog*
- *Debugging*
- *Deleting the Personal*
- *The Finest Four-Letter Word —
  Work!*

The old Sugar Loaf country school had only two rooms for all eight grades. I was one of three eighth graders in the "big room." Slate boards lined the walls. They constituted our bulletin board, billboard, overhead projector, TV, and computer screen all in one. Everything public went on them — tests, outlines, teacher talks, our figuring.

As the week progressed, lots of material remained up there: new spelling and vocabulary words, math formulas and questions, assignments. Gradually the "use and erase" portion of the board got smaller and smaller, and by Friday we not only had limited work space, we also lived in fear of accidentally erasing "something important." That board got ugly, complicated, and patchy, with twenty different little "do not erase" jottings scattered about.

It must have been my "clean genes" rallying to my future profession, because four o'clock Friday was my favorite hour. Miss Rickets would give us the signal and we got to *erase everything!* The chalk dust flew, revealing in all its gray splendor a clean slate — room for a future! Arriving on Monday morning to a clean slate was so much more magical than trudging in on Wednesday or Thursday, and especially on Friday, when the board seemed to sag from dozens of assignments and rules.

I remember going to a school where they had no Friday erasing party and the board was always filled solid and the students and teachers had to write in teeny-weeny letters to squeeze anything in. How perfectly this parallels our office situation. Lots of us have no Friday: our commitments and unfinished tasks all get left "hanging," leaving no room for anything else.

Why Clean Counts

Operating with a clean slate makes work simple in two great ways:

- Physically: It gives us the actual R-O-O-M to put and place things (not to mention the room to work)!

- Mentally: Think about all the positive feelings the idea of "space" conjures up — crisp, fresh, uncluttered, spacious ROOM.

❖ ❖ ❖ ❖

Things that linger get fragmented, forgotten. Worst of all, when something new, bigger, and better comes along, our slate is so full we can't capture it; we have no room for it atop our desks, on our schedules, or in our minds. Ironically, leftover "slated stuff" is often small stuff, simple, easy things that we put off until later and later still. Most of these things we can easily do, and we do really want to get them done:

- Letters to answer
- Calls to return
- Forms to fill out
- Recommendations to review
- Bills to pay
- Things to order
- Things to read
- Things to get fixed

This book can't cover all the whys, whens, wheres, whats, and hows of clearing your slate, but you can do it with no book at all. Just pop into a new policy of erasing your board every Friday afternoon or Saturday morning. Or go even further: clean your slate daily so you can show up the next day and work *ahead,* rather than behind.

Don't get me wrong. Sure, we all have projects, jobs, and obligations that carry over from one day or week to the next. It's the erasable things we should and can do now, easily and inexpensively. So let's rid ourselves of them and start the office week with a clean slate that's waiting to be filled up with all those fresh and exciting new things!

END-OF-WEEK CLEAN SLATE CHECKLIST

❑ Transfer all notes from scattered scraps of paper and jottings to a master list.

❑ Catch up on as many calls as possible, even if it means making some from home.

❑ Get rid of any obvious clutter and junk, such as unneeded copies and trash or recyclables.

❑ Do up next week's list. (You'll be better focused on Monday.)

❑ Process the mail — totally.

❑ Tell others what you have scheduled for next week.

❑ Firm up anything that's unsure or unclear (appointments, assignments, etc.).

❑ Pack up, stack up, or make a list of anything you're going to use next week.

❑ While you're at it, wipe the slate clean of grudges, grievances, and the other mental clutter.

Doing Things Now

Our office battery still holds a charge, it's just dead when certain "staller" items come along, those things we put off, dread, don't do:

- Filling out expense accounts and reports
- Typing up the notes we took
- Holding that negative personnel evaluation session
- Telling the boss we aren't going to be able to make the company picnic
- Honoring that lunch date with Wendell Weary
- Committing to a time for our annual company physical
- Going through those old, old files

We *know* these things need doing, but we've managed to push them to the side. We've been stalling for weeks, months, suffering over them, but so far our efforts in their direction have amounted to 100 percent pure avoidance. To date, we've probably lost thirty hours of productive time, worrying about them, magnifying them in our minds, and shuffling them from list to list. We've faced every way but up to them, putting them off, waiting and hoping for a rescue, hoping some office knight will step in and do them for us.

Procrastinating is like ignoring an aching tooth — it only gets worse and costs more the longer we delay. Right now, we could probably do every single one of the things on our lists in about half a day. But the longer we wait, the more complications develop and the more time they'll ultimately absorb. Soon, those four hours will become eight and then sixteen hours of calls and requests and explanations and more notes and demands and to-dos.

So let's do things now, even the "dreaders," before they have a chance to expand and develop complications and gather "interest" that we will have to pay. Some of these things will take only five or ten minutes to do, once we finally commit ourselves to the doing!

Clearing That Backlog

We're behind, we have a backlog, an overload, an overwhelming mass piled up and more coming. Where do we start? First, remember that we worked our way into this, so we can work our way out.

❖ ❖ ❖ ❖

Facing a "too full" office is about the same as jumping into a cold lake for a swim. We know it's going to be a shock, but the longer we hold back or just dip a toe in to test the water, the harder it gets to take the plunge. But once we do jump in and get going with great enthusiasm (real or simulated), it isn't bad.

Backlogs grow more mentally than they do physically. We lose heart when we just start pecking away at a few things, and then hit a snag and see that looming pile. Instead, let's *launch* ourselves at it. Then watch it shrink.

Try the following battle plan:

1. Orient and assign. Simply pick up every single piece or batch of paper and take a good look at it. At least half of the pile is junk — obsolete or unneeded stuff. Trash the trash, pass the stuff that belongs somewhere else, store the store-worthy,

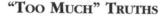

"Too Much" Truths

If you need some incentive, here are a few basic truths about "too much":

• Forever having to rummage and paw through piles constitutes ugly self-punishment.

• A big, invisible speaker hangs over your work space broadcasting one of two messages to your colleagues, clients, customers, and the boss: "I'm in control, I have things together," or: "OUT OF CONTROL!"

• The mess isn't going to vanish by itself. It'll only get worse if you leave it this way.

• No one else can do this for you. At the very least, you have to sort through it all, after which you may discover that other people can execute or dispose of items for you.

• Even if you clean it up once, it will come back again if you don't correct the habits that create it.

and create a "To Do Now" pile. Stack in the second pile the letters that don't need answers right away; reports that can be studied at leisure; and interesting advertisements, offers, and magazines. You can deal with that second pile at a less stressful time.

Wading through it all should provide a clear sense of what's going on, of what to do now and what to do later. Plus — a biggie — the tough things you run into while scouring the stack will be simmering in your mind while you complete the diddly work. You'll have answers and shortcuts ready before you face the difficult items. Also, during this first pass, if you hit a headachy piece of work on which you could use some help, you can call or ask for it right then, and toss the toughie on the "later" pile, where it can await help's arrival.

2. Now take about an hour on the fullest desk or table and reduce the piles and poundage to a respectable-looking load. If you find anything big and easy that you can get out of the way quickly, do it first. There's something very motivating about having the heft of the backlog reduced.

3. While engrossed in this clearing of the clutter, you'll undoubtedly spot more stuff sneaking in through the door or mail slot. Sort it the same way, don't set it aside to tackle after you've banished the backlog. Often, the bulk of these things have an instant solution or can be turned around right away, whereas letting them lay may end up costing you a three-hour marathon.

4. In the end, you probably won't get everything done. So take at least part of it with you, on that business trip, to lunch, or on vacation. Amazing how quick a carried pile (and those magazines) will disappear! You can knock it off while traveling, waiting for your entrée, or enduring TV commercials.

De-bugging

De-bugging is a great simplifier! We aren't talking about ants or cockroaches here, either. Very few of us are truly "laid back" — things can easily bug us around the office:

- The temperature (too hot or too cold)
- The smallness of our office
- No storage for all the stuff they expect us to do
- Poor janitorial services
- Bad parking facilities
- His Tootsie Pops or her gum
- The radio that's constantly blasting
- Slow elevators

❖ ❖ ❖ ❖

It's scary how we can (and will) shift our focus from our job or assignment to distractions like these, stomping and stewing over them instead of focusing on our real objective. Of course, some of these really *are* "buggers." If we've hated them all our lives we can't ignore them or gain instant immunity. When something really bugs us (especially gum popping!), it makes work miserable, and our productivity plummet. Simply put, work isn't simple anymore.

❖ ❖ ❖ ❖

Whining and complaining doesn't get us anywhere. We get told, "You are the only one it bothers," "The boss's kids do the janitorial work," or "We all love Hank's music." So pick one or more of the alternatives here for successful debugging:

1. Inform offenders that their habit bothers you. Many don't realize it and will cease and desist.
2. Move yourself, or ask to be moved, to a more private area, even an ugly one, where you can escape the irritation.
3. Wear earplugs or a headset.
4. Discuss the "bugging" problem with the boss and let him or her face down the do-badders.
5. Figure out a creative way to overcome the things that can't be changed, such as that slow elevator. (For instance, decide to take the stairs and race it.)
6. Quit the job! Enough bugs may merit it. Some workplaces (the conditions, the pay, the language used there, etc.) are simply intolerable.

Don't battle what bugs you, beat it!

Deleting the Personal

Of course we all bring our personal problems to work. They're with us always and everywhere, a part of us — the more severe, the more likely to affect our work. The lesser ones we can and should make a conscious effort to keep out of our minds and thinking once we cross that office threshold. This can be a real relief, to have at least eight hours of the day free from wondering or worrying about them.

❖ ❖ ❖ ❖

Our personal problems can spread like measles: we can contaminate half the staff with them. So before we sit down at the computer, we should clear our mental circuits of minor personal preoccupations.

❖ ❖ ❖ ❖

As for the big ones, the ones we can't get out of our minds or banish, we simply have to try to stay aware of how much they're diverting our attention, and compensate. Somewhere in that office sits a jealous master who pays us for a whole-hearted, not an aching-hearted, effort. So whatever time we lose over such matters (and we're the only ones who really know) should be made up, by coming in early, working late, putting in a Saturday or two. We all deserve the generosity of others when life-shattering experiences befall us, but continually carrying around crises courts disaster.

Top Secret

Private, secret, personal stuff pops up around an office all the time. The government puts its privacies in a big brown envelope provocatively stamped "for ____ eyes only." I used to keep all my "secret" records in a drawer marked: "This is proprietary information pertinent only to me. In case of my demise, just destroy all contents of this drawer."

The drawer contained records of promises I'd made, intimate intelligence people shared with me, information about who cheated and who didn't pay. One day I said to myself, "Really, who, even my closest business partners and dearest family, is going to honor my request to ditch this stuff unread? It'll get read before my will and the cash value of my insurance policy."

I decided that drawerful wasn't worth the risk to me or the reputations of others. So one day I just dumped it, and I felt good. I lost a big worry by clearing this particular slate.

I realize, of course, that most employees will never, *should* never, have even a single folder full of such stuff. However, it's a rare person who has *nothing* similar squirreled away. What should we do with it, then? If anything there is absolutely vital to the company, turn it over to them. Trash the rest. Clear the slate by forgiving and forgetting.

The Finest Four-Letter Word — Work!

An important part of that clear slate we've targeted is our attitude toward the work we do every day. Too often we unthinkingly assign work unfavorable connotations. Homework, housework, yard work, office work, paperwork, book work, catchup work — they all suggest drudgery, toil, slogging, and grinding. Daddy and Mommy have to go to work, you kids have to do your schoolwork, and on Saturday we have to do the housework. Pretty dreary outlook on things, eh? We too easily forget that in bad times people beg and fight to get work. Instead we relegate work to the oppressive "got to," "have to" part of living. And then we spend hours, weeks, and years thinking, scheming, and saving to get out of it. We sue, whine, demand, and stretch our vacations and "sick" days. And this despite air-conditioned offices, huge salaries, and all kinds of privileges, breaks, and benefits.

❖ ❖ ❖ ❖

Maybe we should ask ourselves why we work. To make a living, to survive? To make enough money to get something we want or need? To finance our retirement? Actually, the happiest and most successful people I know, many of whom don't have to work at all, still work their tails off ten or twelve hours a day. Because it's *fun*. They've ignored all the labels, avoided most of the needless burdens, simplified things, and found the gem of accomplishment. And they treasure it.

W hile I was writing one of my recent books, *How to Have a 48-Hour Day,* another one called *Work a Four-Hour Day* appeared on the market. Many acquaintances told me "People don't want a forty-eight-hour day, Don, they want less work." That disagrees with all the people I hear daily murmuring, begging, and even praying for "more time." More time for what? To get more done. More what done? More work, which is the label for about ninety percent of our worthwhile activities, from needlework to teamwork to garden work to artwork.

❖ ❖ ❖ ❖

T hrough years of observation I've come to realize that it's seldom the work itself that people don't like or really dread, because most work can be tremendously rewarding. It's all that other stuff that pollutes this royal four-letter word — equipment problems, technology intimidation, the reports, the waiting, the lines, the taxes, the time clocks, competition, the politics, the smoke, the noise, and on and on. Most people really love work in its purer sense, when and if they can manage to simplify things and just do it. This book tries to suggest some filters to strain those chores and goals and jobs through, so you can rediscover how precious work is when it is simply... just work. What we want to avoid is not the work, but the garbage, the "too much," that spoils our pleasure in working. Pure work is wonderful, so let's eliminate the ugly, unnecessary complications.

2

Conquering the Clock

In this chapter . . .

- *Clock-Watching*
- *Minimizing Interruptions*
- *No-Count Contact*
- *"Late"*
- *Attending to Business*
- *Scheduling*
- *Juggling Priorities*
- *Multitracking*
- *Trimming the To-Dos*

Work would be simple if I had enough time." "We are out of time." "Just give me another hour a day and..." "The deadline!"

We're all obsessed with "time" these days, but time is neutral, we don't really control its passing. We don't stretch it, shrink it, or even manage it — we just use it. We can only control conditions, not clocks.

I did a "get more done" seminar for a large school system not long ago. As a warm-up exercise, all of the participants were asked to divide a circle into wedges representing how they spent, organized, and scheduled their time. Then one by one they explained their division.

The eye-opening consensus was — overload! Absolutely no room to fit anything else in! They all felt frustrated about the absent slice — "time for me" or time for that special project or time to perform community service. Most of them lived for the day when they could cut out one of the activities and squeeze the really important one into the circle.

We all know that won't happen — there's no more time later on. Actually, we get busier as we get more experienced and efficient and able. The more we can do, the more we take on. And the more others add on (consider that a compliment!).

❖ ❖ ❖ ❖

So what are our options? Crowd (a stress and pressure procedure), or change things around and redivide that pie! Assuming that our established slices must be adopted permanently is the error of our office (and home) ways. We don't have to accept every one of our present activities and the time, money, and emotion they take.

Routine robs our time more than anything else. We must continually shake down our schedule, goals, and project lists, until we can replace an unproductive wedge of our "pie" with a satisfying portion of things that really matter.

Clock-Watching

Watching the clock is always bad news. It reveals that our heart isn't in the job, only in getting relief from it. Those constant glances upward don't impress others, either.

❖ ❖ ❖ ❖

Two people helped cure me of clock-watching:

- My seventh-grade teacher, having noticed my intense interest in the big timepiece hanging above George Washington, handed me a slip of paper that said: "Time will pass. Will you?"
- Another friend, years later, suggested that a clock was for racing, not watching. Thus I discovered the fun of beating the clock, of seeing how much I could get done, how fast, before time ran out.

❖ ❖ ❖ ❖

To avoid the "What time is it?" syndrome, we can be *early.* That way we don't have to measure minutes or feel stress over seconds.

❖ ❖ ❖ ❖

The best way of all to avoid clock-watching (a.k.a. wishing away your life) is to switch, or get ourselves switched, to something that interests us more. When we're truly interested in what we're doing, we look at the clock only to see how much time we have left to work on it.

Minimizing Interruptions

"**M**an, I have to get out of the office to get anything done." A sad commentary or sane warning? An office really locates us, pins us down to a spot, so everyone knows where to find us. And indeed they will, at their convenience, call or stop by and chat about even the most piddling thing. Without some real discipline our offices can easily become social centers instead of work centers. Such interruptions and distractions make us lose focus. Instead of taking bites out of our daily workload, we nibble crumbs. It's been estimated that it takes about twenty minutes to really get into something, so constant stops and restarts really take their toll. The cure?

1. Close the door, ask someone to take messages, and post a "Do Not Disturb" sign.
2. Use seven hours of the office day to concentrate on the actual work and one hour — in one chunk — to meet, eat, exchange, talk, and expedite. Sure, immediates and emergencies crop up, forcing us to drop everything else, but not as many of them as we imagine.
3. Even if the office opens at 9:00, don't open *your* office — take any calls or visitors — until 10:00. This frees an undisturbed hour to get it all together: plan, organize, review that important matter or report, make important calls.
4. Set up a second, "quiet" office. I work at home early, early, for four or five hours to get the "closed door" work done. Then I use my public office for public work.

❖ ❖ ❖ ❖

"This will just take a minute" usually means at least fifteen minutes. Give the one minute and make an appointment for the other fourteen.

To gain some quiet and uninterrupted time without working more than forty hours: if your job allows this flexibility, set up a very different kind of schedule one or two days a week. On those days, come in very early and leave early, or come in late and stay late.

❖ ❖ ❖ ❖

Avoid surprises. Surprises are for parties, not the workplace. Anything unexpected means something we're unprepared for. The unscheduled can and will occur, but usually at a cost greater than that of the scheduled.

❖ ❖ ❖ ❖

Unavoidable interruptions will happen. So allow for them, don't flip out. Instead, relax and try to enjoy the interruption as a change of pace.

❖ ❖ ❖ ❖

If interruptions happen too often, investigate whether you're overbooked, planning poorly, or being taken advantage of.

❖ ❖ ❖ ❖

Cut down on the fiddling with food. Nothing interrupts, or distracts, like the appearance of home-made brownies or seven-topping pizzas. At least 85 percent of us are overfed already, but we all flock to the spread, spreading crumbs and sticky stuff all over. And then we end up feeling sluggish and lazy for hours afterward.

No-Count Contact

Should we jump every time anyone yells "Frog!"? At work, where ten thousand agendas surround us and instant communication abounds, things just as nonsensical are yelled at us daily. We get calls and letters from salespeople of all kinds, invitations to everything imaginable, appeals and requests by the bundle. How much of this deserves to go on our schedule or to-do list, for callback or reply?

Deciding what merits our response is a judgment call only we can make. Courtesy and professionalism require that we acknowledge and respond to sincere and thoughtful contacts. But I have several calls a day, for example, from brokers with "a deal for me." I've told them I'm not interested, several times, and still they call, so I ignore with a clear conscience.

❖ ❖ ❖ ❖

Hard-boiled businesses cut off the stream of questionable solicitations long ago — publishing, for example, with the little notation "no unsolicited manuscripts" and the movie business, by the requirement "through registered agents only."

❖ ❖ ❖ ❖

Often, one kindly response or encouragement on our part generates an endless succession of communications that lead nowhere, as far as our professional agenda is concerned. We all have to find and stick to a sensible and ethical response policy, or we'll be buried.

"Late"

When we're late on anything, even a little late, we touch off a chain reaction that can affect hundreds of people and cost thousands of dollars. Offices organize and conduct things according to a schedule. Schedule violations — someone doesn't show, the package doesn't come, the check is late, the meal is late, the flight is late — force everyone to immediately adjust. This can mean scores of calls and interruptions, do-overs and redos, reschedulings and cancellations.

❖ ❖ ❖ ❖

We often joke about, apologize for, and justify "Late," but one way or another it always gets punished. To complicate our own work or sabotage a competitor, nothing succeeds like "Late." Late is also the winner in the confidence-reducing derby.

❖ ❖ ❖ ❖

What's the biggest cause of "Late"? That's easy — it's *starting* late! Think about it.

> *"Late" is an act of dishonesty that robs its victims of time, money, and emotional reserves.*

Attending to Business

Many who find work complicated, complicate it more by spotty attendance, and when you're not there to handle problems as they arise, small problems can become large very quickly.

ABSENCE ADDS UP

We all underestimate the impact of absence caused by, for example, geting out of bed late or having to tend to personal matters on company time. I know an executive in the upper management of a company who constantly tells me he never takes any personal time or vacation even though he's entitled to three weeks a year. Yet I notice the single days or half days he takes off regularly for various personal activities. That's only three or four days a month, hardly noticeable, but by the time the end of the year rolls around, it adds up to forty-two days, or six weeks off a year! People do notice, and most businesspeople can count.

Little streams fill raging rivers, and minor time misses can add up to an avalanche of absence.

Be tough on talking. We all like talking about 300 percent more than listening, and work seems the perfect place to exercise our jawbone. Consider that innocent thing called chitchatting. We do it at the fountain, over the copy machine, in the office doorway, and on personal calls. When six or eight people meet in the hall to discuss someone's new haircut, imagine how much that haircut has cost the company. Forget the hair and cut the chatter instead.

❖ ❖ ❖ ❖

If we chitchat five minutes of every hour, that's the best part of an hour a day lost "visiting." Add that three-quarters of an hour back into our actual work time, and it may do a lot to cover the need for "more help in the office."

Shooting the breeze has shot down more profits than any fluctuation in the market

Scheduling

It's best to use only one central calendar for tracking all events, meetings, and obligations, including personal ones that may have a bearing on our work lives. Having more than one scheduling calendar is just asking for things to be overlooked — you'll forget to transfer them, or put them on one and not the other!

❖ ❖ ❖ ❖

Your calendar should be the most accessible thing on your desk, the easiest thing to grab. And keep any backup references right by it.

Belonging Blues

The workplace seems to attract associations and organizations of all kinds — professional, community minded, and service oriented. But there are more fellowships, fraternities, orders, societies, leagues, and brother- and sisterhoods than you can count. True, many of them are worthwhile. Even more true, they all want good souls like us to join. So what should we do?

Pick carefully and join sparingly. Hold the line on "belonging," or you'll wake up someday to find yourself overcommitted and overcommitteed, with half your time, energy, and emotion going into preparing for and attending meetings. We all want to come through once we've accepted responsibility, and fulfilling the obligations and requests of a half-dozen clubs or associations is far from simple.

The simple moral: It may sound impressive to be the king, queen, or jack-of-all-trade associations, but the work realm suffers.

A corollary: Unencumbered is still the ace of "simple."

❖ ❖ ❖ ❖

If you or your manager has an appointment calendar that several people need to consult, consider entering appointments and meetings by typing them out on little stick-on labels. It's much easier and safer than everyone trying to decipher things scribbled there in cramped and illegible handwriting. Better still, purchase scheduling software.

❖ ❖ ❖ ❖

Rule number one for appointments: Crowd the morning! Schedule things for the morning, especially the early hours. This works for you in four ways:

1. It forces you to prepare the day before.
2. Morning appointments will be briefer. Many people start out behind schedule or "have to get somewhere."
3. It frees the rest of the day.
4. "Early" weeds out the weak who may otherwise waste your time.

❖ ❖ ❖ ❖

The worst appointment time is anywhere around lunchtime (eleven o'clock to two o'clock). That's when people are always late (because of traffic, for example), paying too much attention to their rumbling stomachs, or coming down with a case of the after-lunch yawns.

❖ ❖ ❖ ❖

On calendars, make a clear distinction between the definite and the iffy, between, for example, "hold" and "confirmed" dates. And the minute something is confirmed, be sure to change it to confirmed!

Juggling Priorities

Lists. Love them and don't lose them! You can make work simple by doing just two things with lists:

1. Make them.
2. Follow them.

❖ ❖ ❖ ❖

We all have to be our own list makers because only we know what needs to go on them. But let me offer a few list fine-tuners:

- We're often too short-range with our lists. We don't make them far enough into the future, and we wait too long to make them. Notice how many people who make "must lists" for doing or going, do it just prior to actually doing or going. Making that list months, not minutes ahead provides a time cushion for remembering more items and for thinking of ways you can piggyback things, thereby letting them do double duty.
- Make your lists on something consistent — not the backs of envelopes, Post-its, business cards, two-by-fours, the palm of your hand, or the tablecloth. Adopt or adapt a list document or software tool and then use the same format for *all* your lists. That way they're easy to find and keep together. Convert all messages, memos, calls, and notifications to your own format, familiar and easily reorganized.

- Make conversation lists a habit. We've all done project lists, shopping lists, lists of instructions or directions, of places to eat out — you name it, we've done it, and it's done us a lot of good, too. So, why not make a list of what you want to talk about in a call or meeting? We generally do this in our mind but remember only three or four of the six or seven things we wanted to say or ask. I write up a little list before every phone call and it saves callbacks, embarrassment, expensive oversights, and the inevitable (with a slap to the head) "Oh, I forgot!"

❖ ❖ ❖ ❖

Use schedules to organize and moods to prioritize. You'll get more done, faster and better, and enjoy it more. Learning to fly when things flow is a real work simplifier, whereas having to wade and slog often results from not doing things when we were in the mood earlier.

❖ ❖ ❖ ❖

If you set a time to stop work and go home, stick to it.

❖ ❖ ❖ ❖

Schedule "date night" with a friend, spouse, or significant other. Work becomes simpler when home stays happy.

❖ ❖ ❖ ❖

Priorities are personal preferences in the end, neither deadline nor schedule driven.

Multitracking

Doing more than one thing at a time is a skill we grow into. We start life learning to start a job, finish it, then start another, finish it, and so on. This is okay until we reach a point in life and at work where we have more to do and people expect more of us. Our jobs grow more complicated daily, involving ever more people and objectives. Suddenly, single-focus order isn't sufficient any more. We have to do many things at the same time.

The old remark "he can't walk and chew gum at the same time" is a cop-out. He — *we* — not only can walk and chew at the same time, we can also fix, find, think, notice, exercise, carry, help, organize, gather, and write.

❖ ❖ ❖ ❖

Doing more than one thing at a time simply means running on several tracks at once. There is no miracle or magic involved, and not even much might. We can do as many things at once as we want, as long as we don't start or stop more than one thing at the same time.

❖ ❖ ❖ ❖

We can handle all sorts of emergencies and turn all sorts of negatives into positives if we just forget the old one-job-at-a-time routine. The multitrack system takes a little discipline and practice, but most mothers already have it developed to a fine art, which is why many of them re-entering the work force can outmanage the rest of us at least two to one!

❖ ❖ ❖ ❖

There are a lot of little "waits" in office work. The smart thing to do is to make use of them. We can line up some little chores for when we're on hold, talking on the phone to a long-winded person, or waiting for that "I'll call you right back." Or for when the computer is down, printing, or booting up. Some starter ideas: look up addresses, stuff envelopes, label disks, dejunk the middle drawer of your desk, sort through the in-box, make new file folders and label them, proofread letters, make copies, clear obsolete data off your hard drive, update your project list.

SUBORDINATING CONJUNCTIONS

At the office we can always do more than our "A" priorities on any given day, because we have seven big helpers at our disposal:

- *Before* — Before getting to work.
- *After* — After everyone clears out.
- *Whenever* — Whenever we have unexpected downtime.
- *Until* — Until the printout prints.
- *While* — While we eat or wait on hold.
- *Wherever* — Wherever inspiration strikes.
- *Because* — Because we *can* think, organize, and chew gum at the same time

---

Think ahead, try to foresee the next step, plan how to make what you're doing now segue to the next task. Looking ahead will also help you collect everything you need for what comes next.

Trimming the To-Dos

We should deal with things as much as possible the minute we get them in our hands. Read and toss, read and file, read and put it wherever else it belongs. In other words, don't just pile things up.

Likewise, when something new crops up, and it's not a big thing, don't "prioritize" it and put it in a pile of things to do later, because it may take forever to get back to it. Stop and do it right then. Otherwise, your "undone" will undo you.

❖ ❖ ❖ ❖

Subordinates aren't the only ones we can delegate to, we can also delegate to peers and bosses. Some of the most successful delegation is sideways. Many things can be better handled by someone with more clout or a different position.

❖ ❖ ❖ ❖

What can we do to remedy a badly overworked, understaffed situation, or a dynamic, growing one, with far too many "to-dos" to ever get to? One possibility is the "squeaky wheel" approach.

If your department handles largely in-house requests, where public PR isn't much of an issue, you can set priorities largely by follow-up. If someone cares enough about something to actually follow up on it, it must be important to them or actually needed. If no follow-up follows, keep it on the "B" list.

You can even wait for a *second* follow-up, but this is risky. If someone follows up twice, it's definitely important to them, but it may be too late to do them any good. Wait too long, and you get no credit for doing the job. And the blame lands on you if something falls through because it sat for two and a half months in your in-basket.

TAKING THE HEAT

If you have an incredibly long project list, you can try a bold approach. This may not work for everyone, but it will do wonders in the right situations.

Pick the half-dozen hottest projects, the "big stuff" that would mean the most to the company or department in terms of growth and profits. Move them to the top of your list and never work on anything else unless you can't advance any of the top six for some reason. Leave everything else on a B list, without deadlines.

This means you must be prepared to take the heat, to let people get annoyed, even your supervisor. This will be hard at first, because we usually want to fulfill requests, especially when an authority figure makes them. But try to be stoic. Week to week people may jump on you about removing the scuffs on the wall or designing the program for next year's company playlet. But when it comes time for your performance review (and raises and promotions), they'll remember that you made the company two million dollars, not that you didn't finish writing the proofreaders' manual.

Accomplish the hundred-thousand-dollar tasks and, no matter how irritated they are, people won't take you to serious task for the nickel-and-dime stuff.

Some office projects and assignments (yes, even ones from your manager) may not have been carefully thought out.

If you disagree with a particular assignment, don't just accept it, challenge the sense or priority of it, right there and then, or at least make the boss defend its priority. Better to take heat for challenging it right then, than to agree to do it and then not come through.

If your supervisor ends up agreeing with you, terrific. Together, maybe the two of you can find another way to accomplish the goal.

3

The Office Ecosystem

In this chapter . . .

- *Our Workstation*
- *Windows and Lights*
- *Designing and Remodeling*
- *Getting Comfortable*

When we go camping, where and how we set up camp controls how comfortable our wilderness headquarters will be. If we pitch our tent near a swamp, on a hillside, or in a dry creek bed, we can inflict as much distraction upon the experience as setting up our office workplace in the middle of traffic, in a dark, crowded cubbyhole, or under the building loudspeaker.

Our work setting constitutes our inside ecosystem, and we want to plant ourselves, our furnishings, and the tools of our trade for maximum convenience, efficiency, and comfort. Anything we have to fight will gradually render us inefficient and forever fidgety.

Our Workstation

Unless we're in a business where a sharp appearance is part of what we're selling, let's leave the fancy offices to the egoists. "Overdecorated" and "overfurnished" are only a distraction. Expensive handmade rugs, collectibles, and objects of art — stainable, stealable, and breakable — only complicate things. Ogling them, showing them off, polishing them, and worrying about them does nothing for either communication or concentration.

The trappings don't matter much. Just give me some square footage to spread out my work, a phone nearby, a thick door, a long to-do list, and a big wastebasket.

An old fifty-dollar office salvage desk has served many a successful millionaire, while mahoganymania has mustered out many a megalomaniac.

Ever notice all the energy and planning (if not scheming) that go into picking or assigning a place for an office? — a frenzy of "keep me out of the basement" or "I want a window." Most people covet the power positions, such as a corner or an alcove, but we're better off leaving the vain to claim those spots. More important, if we have any choice at all in the matter, we should avoid the following *bad* places:

- Near any door, especially an outside door, where you'll fight cold and heat, noise, and the wind blowing things off the desk and walls
- Next to the copier
- Along the traffic lanes, where everyone stops to say hello and people talk over, around, or behind you (you won't be able to think straight or hear the phone)
- Where anyone who walks by can see what's on your computer screen
- Right by a bathroom or break room
- Directly underneath an air-conditioning or heating vent
- In a window

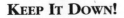

KEEP IT DOWN!

Some people can work amidst noise and distraction, in fact they seem to need action, movement, music around them. Many others need quiet — even a tiny hum bothers them. If you like rap music and a coworker hates it, try earphones. If those rattling pipes drive you crazy, try earplugs.

Soft floor and wall coverings, thick walls, acoustic ceilings, and solid-core doors do a lot to muffle sound. Sound-absorbing window coverings can help, too, though here we may have to balance the issue of noise reduction against the desirability of natural light.

Windows and Lights

These days, the primary value of windows is prestige, as the modern-day HVACs (interior air-handling systems) do even better when it comes to ventilation than an open window did in the old days. And an interesting view out the window may even be more of a distraction than an aid to office work, especially if it's a floor-to-ceiling window and people constantly walk by (and peer in).

❖ ❖ ❖ ❖

Windows have many drawbacks. Chilly drafts, for one. Plus, direct sunlight and heat are bad for computers, and a window behind your computer screen will cause eyestrain as your eyes try to adjust to two different levels of light at the same time. You'll be looking into glare, and at night passing car lights may plague you.

❖ ❖ ❖ ❖

If you are shorted a window and it really bothers you:

- Hang up an attractive painting or poster of the outdoors.
- Paper one wall of the office with something that lifts your spirits, maybe even a photo mural.
- Paint one wall light blue, with a few dabs of fluffy cloud.
- Put colorful curtains over an imaginary window.

As for lights, first turn them on. We often see people squinting when a nearby bank of handy lights is sitting there waiting for someone to hit the switch.

❖ ❖ ❖ ❖

Lighting is the most economical use of energy out there! If you can't see at work, don't just put up with it; see that an eye-friendly new unit is added to your station. Don't fight poor light — especially in the home office, where all too many of us operate in the dark. Enough light is a wonderful simplifier.

Designing and Remodeling

When we're planning or remodeling an office, the first thing we need to do is sit down and make a list of every piece of equipment we own, and every piece we plan to purchase. We need to know lengths, widths, heights, and sometimes weights, plus how far from the wall things will stick out. Even if it may be a couple of years before a purchase is made, we need to allow space for it. Measure, measure, measure!

❖ ❖ ❖ ❖

You don't have to be an artist or an architect to draw a rough layout of how you want your office to work. If necessary, make little paper cutouts (to the right scale) of furniture and equipment and then shuffle them around on a piece of graph paper.

A key question: Where do the phone and electric lines come in? Be sure you know where the equipment is going to be, so you can have the proper jacks and outlets, and enough of them. Most standard outlets are 110 volts, but some equipment calls for 220.

❖ ❖ ❖ ❖

Leave enough wall space for bulletin boards, chalkboards, or other "wall work spaces." Make sure the wall is available, accessible, and not blocked from view.

❖ ❖ ❖ ❖

Plan for storage, too — don't let it be an afterthought. Knowing your storage requirements is essential to any well-run business. Well-organized storage areas can make or break you.

Don't forget to allow for growth.

Getting Comfortable

An uncomfortable office layout is a big deterrent to progress. We shouldn't fight furniture and fixtures that are hard to work on or around, the wrong height, depth, or weight, or just plain inconvenient.

Make sure your work area fits you — you don't want a desk too high or one you crack your knees on. Alter and adapt your office to fit you — anything that's in the way or too far away, change it now, today. If you're too short, tall, big, or little to fit the counter, table, desk, or chair, or to reach the files or the mirror or the light, adjust or replace them. Suffering by using "what's available" is not simple by the end of a long day. So block up, saw off, glue on, add wheels, or whatever, but fit things to you.

- Move to a handy location those files you need to grab when the phone rings.
- Hang the phone on the wall if it takes up too much room on the desk.
- Raise file cabinets that are too low.
- Use the file drawer that's too high for storage.
- Put a trash can where trash is generated, not where it looks best.
- Get rid of pictures that distract or depress you.
- Add or subtract plants or photos that help or hurt the mood.
- Add signs, labels, longer cords, a table, or whatever will ease and enhance what you're doing.

❖ ❖ ❖ ❖

If you're left-handed and everything (tools, layouts) is set up for the right-hander, change things to fit you. It will only take a tiny bit of time and expense now, but save you years of physical strain and mental aggravation.

Be sure to arrange things to save steps — have the printer close to the computer, the printing supplies near the printer, the file cabinets near the desk, if you do your own filing. Constantly getting up to retrieve things is annoying, and we're all too likely to get distracted in the process.

❖ ❖ ❖ ❖

One heavy-duty electric cord bank (breaker) in a central location saves having extension cords snaking to every outlet in the room.

❖ ❖ ❖ ❖

Don't worry about "standard desk furnishings." Keep only what *you* really use on your desktop. If you never use a tape dispenser, dispense with it! Move out that fancy pen set and blotter if all they do is collect dust. Ditto those paperweights if they never weight paper.

❖ ❖ ❖ ❖

Clear working space is a real luxury and a high, so don't sacrifice it to things you don't really care about or haven't used in years. Take a hard look at everything on your desktop today.

❖ ❖ ❖ ❖

Although space (or the office "decorating code") often limits what personal touches you can add to an office, they're still important. A small family portrait, a drawing from your child, or just a card from a loved one allows you to claim your area as your own.

Choose an office clock that's attractive and quiet, and place it where it's easy for all to see.

❖ ❖ ❖ ❖

Plants in the office: Too often they end up a sad, scraggly remnant of that lush greenery we started with. So confine yourself to plants with a fighting chance of flourishing in an office setting, ones that thrive under artificial light and take well to pruning. Ask a florist or consult a houseplant guide. Take ill-suited gift plants home so they can have a window, or find them a new home.

❖ ❖ ❖ ❖

Visiting children: One attorney keeps a small table covered with books, coloring books and crayons, and drawing paper for children to amuse themselves while the parents are meeting and talking. The lobby of another office contains a large, attractive basket stuffed with stuffed animals. The office manager explained that these were excellent for visiting children because they didn't make any noise and were easy to pick up afterward. They even had a calming effect on some of the adult visitors to the office.

4

Working Free of Clutter

In this chapter . . .

- *Tending to the Personal*
- *Dealing with the Done*
- *Paper Weight*
- *Elbow Room*
- *Storage*
- *Preventing Future Clutter Now*

I visited an office once where a reporter was reported "not in" and missed two big stories because of it. He was in, but the stacks on his desk had mounted so high that they literally hid him from sight. When he finally dejunked — under "public pressure" — he discovered that almost all of those piles were outdated, worthless paper. Most of us would be equally shocked by a candid list of the contents of our own "workstation."

Let's take a look at a little typical office junk:

- Sixteen unopened introductory offers to try America Online
- *Consumer Report Buying Guide 1992*
- Mug of dried-up markers and pencil stubs
- Box of business cards with the wrong phone number
- One glove left by a visitor (no one remembers when or who)
- Plaque that certifies you were a member of the Chamber of Commerce in 1986
- Manuals to old computer hardware
- Demo videos for equipment you didn't buy
- Corrupted floppy disks
- Little containers of lead in a variety of hardnesses — and you don't even have a mechanical pencil
- Cartridges for a defunct printer

Tending to the Personal

Don't we all want to reform first the world, society, our company, our mate, and only then ourselves? Yet guess what? When and if we clean up and organize ourselves first, many of "their" problems will go away. Most of our junk and clutter problems are personal, so to help make work simple make all those little kingdoms you control yourself clean and orderly. Here's a top-ten list (in no particular order):

1. Your wallet or purse, pockets
2. Your briefcase

3. Your desk drawers
4. Your file cabinets
5. Your stacking trays and desktop
6. Your shelves
7. Your computer's hard disk and your floppy disk collection
8. Your library
9. Your office storage area
10. Your car

Amazing the influence this will have on others, and the whole workplace, too.

❖ ❖ ❖ ❖

Your best office friend is, of course, that wonderful center top desk drawer, so treat it appropriately. It's the mechanic's tool box of our business, holding everything from vital hardware to things we need to hide quickly. Too often, we pay it no mind until it won't close any more. Then we find something important we crammed in there and forgot, or, worse, we can't find anything. Remember, this is an active space, not idle storage. I cured mine of clutter by opening it during those listen-to-a-line phone conversations; I dejunked, culled, reorganized, condensed, and clipped out as I talked. When I was done I tossed out a pile of useless paper and at least three pounds of rusty paper clips, ossified erasers, homeless pen caps, and non-functioning pens. (I'll leave it to you to add drawer dividers or organizers, or small shallow boxes, if you think they will help.)

At home we're each now producing about four pounds of trash per day. One wonders how much we pile up at work for others to dispose of. Together, we and the people at the desks around us generate bushels of trash daily, yet we only seem to clear it away weekly, monthly, or — I can testify to the truth of this — annually. Instead, move any trash off your work space (desk, table, bench, floor, vehicle) daily!

❖ ❖ ❖ ❖

Recyling is the doctrine of the day. Do it willingly and it will quickly become part of your personal code. The office and the environment will be the better for it.

Dealing with the Done

What if you went to the hospital and found that the doctors and nurses only cleaned up every so often, and under the tables and in the corners were old used bandages, cast-off casts, used needles, ancient X rays, replaced heart valves, bone fragments, and other discarded body parts. You'd be horrified, and your image of this place would really suffer. This is exactly what happens with *our* workplace when we let the finished and done with remain around.

❖ ❖ ❖ ❖

The second something has served its purpose, it should GO: into the mail, on to the next office, into the file, into the waste can, wherever — but off and away from our "operating table." Sorting through, digging through, shoving aside, climbing over piles of expired stuff is depressing, and a big waste of time. Yet we carelessly let things accumulate to slow us down, irritate us, and make us look bad.

❖ ❖ ❖ ❖

One big, big simplifier in the office is to dispose of junk and waste *now*. When something is empty, spent, gone, broken, or out of favor, don't ease it into extinction, throw it out or recycle it right now. Even the end of the day is too late. Deal with it this hour, and watch your efficiency rise.

Paper Weight

Not too many years ago a big promise was dangled before us: a "paperless society." We all envisioned those piles and stacks being replaced by recordings, computer screen communications, codes, and the like. Now that we're approaching the millennium, what's the reality? Where we would have had twenty tons of paper per office before, now we have only fifteen. Paper is still burying the office workplace, and it happens so subtly, like:

- Most businesses had one or two professional magazines years ago; today, five to twenty or more.
- Bills for utilities once came on a card. Now every billing envelope contains several pieces of paper.

- The fax (with cover page) generates between two and eight pieces of paper for one simple message.
- The number of catalogs of all kinds has at least quadrupled in the last few years.
- The number of coupons, flyers, brochures, and broadsides has increased at least tenfold due to easier distribution.

OUR FAVORITE PAPER PILE MANEUVER

Pile things up as you go through the day, sorting, dealing with, receiving, and dispatching things. It's OK because every piece of paper that comes in doesn't have a priority that matches the demands at hand. So setting things aside for a later or better time is great.

But take the pile with you when you leave. Don't leave piles of "to-dos" on your desk. They only get bigger and more intimidating. When you take them with you, you'll find all kinds of opportunities to dispose of them, either by doing or by dumping.

So get a big briefcase! When it gets too full you *have to* deal with the pile, which is good for you, good for the pile, and good for those affected by the pile.

We easily can have more than a hundred pages of paper a day to deal with, unless we're in a paper-intensive business, in which case we'll have more. Pitch that excess paper!

❖ ❖ ❖ ❖

Two magic words for decluttering: *Cancel it!* (the subscription, the membership, the credit card).

❖ ❖ ❖ ❖

Studies have shown that at least eighty percent of the stuff in the average paper file never gets used or looked at again. Most of the paper yellowing there is obsolete, outdated, duplicated, a waste of expensive file cabinet space. And if it's unnecessary, it's punishing us, obscuring and confusing things, causing losses, wrong filing, digging, hunting — mistakes and inefficiencies of all kinds. Face up to it soon and I'll bet you can reduce it all to about a third of its present bulk. (Also check the hints under the "Filing" header in Chapter 8, "Keeping Things Moving.")

Elbow Room

All desk jockeys desire "more room" to work, and that would seem an easy problem to solve. Just get a Texas or Alaska desktop! Given our pack rat proclivities, however, our work space will soon be reduced to about the size of one yellow pad and two elbows, regardless of desk size.

Even if you have thirty projects under way, find another place to park all but the one or two that you're working on right now. No need to have twenty-eight others right under your nose or elbows, where they'll only distract you.

The Rules of More Room

- *Rule One:* Use desks only for active projects. Passive or long-range stuff should be moved off the desktop to a drawer or shelf or other surface. Get it out of the way of your daily or weekly traffic.
- *Rule Two:* Make a file folder for everything still lurking on your desk, and then slip the material into the folder. Across the top of the folder, clearly identify the contents. This enables you to stack the folders on their sides, where all the labels show. You can find everything in a second, yet six files only take a small corner of the desk.
- *Rule Three:* Have only one basket on your desk, an in-basket (see Chapter 8).
- *Rule Four:* Remember the janitorial rule: "If the desktop is clear, we clean it. If it's cluttered, we assume it's all personal and important and don't touch it."

As soon as you finish the ones you're working on, or when you've gotten them as far as you can right now, move them off your desk. Use your own system, as we all should, for keeping track of them until they become active again.

❖ ❖ ❖ ❖

As soon as you finish something, get it out of sight and out of the way of the next project!

❖ ❖ ❖ ❖

If you need to clear off your desk and get rid of a particular project for a few weeks, route it to the person who has a reputation for sitting on things, the office black hole or Bermuda Triangle.

Storage

Offices are workstations, not warehouses, museums, or retail outlets. Which means this is not a place for excess stock or souvenirs. We can easily segregate the objects in our offices into two groups, active and passive.

- Keep active things (the stuff you need constantly) in and around your desk.
- Keep passive things (the "need once in a while" stuff) reachable and retrievable but not right with you. This means in a handy storage area, in boxes or containers, that are identified on all four sides and the top. Saves lots of searching and restacking.

Keep things off the floor — things on the floor get wet and get dumped!

❖ ❖ ❖ ❖

It's the millennium, and cardboard (wettable, crushable, insect-attracting cardboard) is obsolete. When you need to store good stuff to do or consult later (much later), use the new jumbo plastic containers, not those old cardboard boxes. These plastic containers come in all sizes, from hand-carrying to cart-hauling size. They look good and are mouse and moisture proof, stackable, and easy to open and close.

Preventing Future Clutter Now

In all its full-color glory, and rife with tantalizing descriptions, the office equipment catalog is almost immoral. Gasp-worthy temptations face us on every page. The *Glamour* magazine of the work site, the equipment catalog presents office props so handy and handsome we just have to have them all. Every fixture and furnishing, aid and accessory imaginable are illustrated here: stands, shelves, racks, holders, trays, sorters, viewers, organizers, clocks, cases, lamps, credenzas, color-coordinated computer workstations Avoid one of the deadliest office sins: avarice. What you didn't know you wanted until you saw it in a catalog, you probably don't really need.

The Computer

In this chapter . . .

I used to wonder how my great-grandfather, who had only a horse and buggy for transportation, would have felt had he lived to see the car invented and developed from a primitive motorized wagon to the luxurious, fully automated speedster of today. But now I know!

In a relatively short period of time, the computer, like the automobile before it, has gone through the stages of initial suspicion on our part, fear of its complexity and power, awe at its image, and astonishment at its offspring. And just as the auto, wonderful as it is, can kill us financially and harm us physically if we don't handle it right, the same is true of the computer. All tools have their trials, and keeping them on our side is serious business.

Computers and ancillary equipment (printers, modems, scanners, and on and on) have become so omnipresent and useful for so many tasks — writing, creating databases and spreadsheets, keeping inventory, projecting schedules, tracking progress, storing all kinds of records, retrieving reference material from the Internet, and even computing! — that some of the basics about how to make their use simpler often get overlooked. Computers are *so* ubiquitous that whole books have been written about using them efficiently in the workplace. (And efficiency is another word for simplicity.) Just look at the expanding catalog of computer books, not to mention the guidebooks that try to simplify (often at upwards of 750 pages!) the instructions in the manuals that come with your software.

Given all the pages of advice out there, anything that we say in this chapter can't help but be dwarfed. And many specific suggestions belong where they'll be most useful to you — for example, some E-mail pointers in Chapter 7 "Corresponding." So what we'll do here is just present a few simple principles and suggestions.

Computer Envy

First, one big beef about computers, accessories, and software (managers, take note): Too often in the office, the people who are going to use the computers and the software aren't consulted in buying them. They're not asked how they like to do things, what projects they have planned, and so forth. And yes, companies often overbuy computers for the wrong people: "He's a vice president, so he needs a fancy computer." The veep may use it once a day, while the assistant who attends all kinds of meetings relies upon a notepad rather than a laptop.

❖ ❖ ❖ ❖

Everyone in most offices doesn't need a dedicated line to the company's Internet server, a gigabyte of memory, 32 megabytes of RAM, and a personal laser printer. Use what you have if it does what you need. Don't waste time and emotional energy coveting the network manager's 200-megahertz behemoth with the 21-inch monitor, 33.6 fax modem, and 16-bit sound system.

❖ ❖ ❖ ❖

If what you have *doesn't* do what you need, don't just gripe. Instead, write up *in detail* what you need, why you need it, and how it will pay off for the company.

For pointers about buying computers and software, take a look at the brief suggestions in Chapter 12, "The Home Office." (They won't pertain to everyone for the obvious reason that most office workers can't just grab an issue of *Computer Shopper* and dial up a toll-free supplier.)

SOFTWARE ETHICS

Many offices buy one copy of a program and copy, copy, copy. Bootlegging is unethical and *illegal*. Face up to it. If you have any say in the matter, pay for a "site license."

Making the Most of Your Electronic Tools

Create an orderly system of directories and subdirectories that make sense to you and your work patterns. Decide on a system for identifying and storing faxes, memos, and files. It also simplifies things if everyone in your office can agree on one system.

❖ ❖ ❖ ❖

Be sure to include footers or headers on printed documents to identify the original's file location and name, as well as the date and time it was printed out. This is especially important for spreadsheets and statistical reports.

Inexpensive programs, such as PCAnywhere, allow you to operate your office computer from home or when traveling, if you have a laptop. You can retrieve, revise, and save your files to either your office or home computer. This saves having to carry disks back and forth, remembering which files you need when, and discovering you have four or five versions of one document to reconcile.

❖ ❖ ❖ ❖

Develop a filing system that uses initial numeric codes that you assign to each project. File all documents related to a specific project in their own subdirectory. For instance, a grant proposal for a community garden might be project number 251. Name its subdirectory "251GARD," and store all documents related to the project there with such names as "251dft", "251ltr1", and so on.

Learning New Software

When learning to use a program, put things you need to remember on index cards, until they're integrated into your daily routine. Saves fishing them out of the giant manual each time. Better still, try using the simple Notepad utility that's included in many software packages, including Microsoft Windows.

Give yourself time to learn how to use new software, to make intuitive leaps. Give yourself the freedom to learn and think, and you may bring new things to the aid of your product and your office work.

❖ ❖ ❖ ❖

Many of the guidebooks now on the market offer valuable shortcuts for streamlining procedures that you use over and over and over. But if you buy or borrow one of these backup books, don't waste time trying to read the whole thing. Your brain will fry. Instead, identify the repetitive task that you want to streamline. Next, try the software's help function, which sometimes is actually helpful. Then, if you need more information, grab the backup book and go immediately to the index — these manuals usually include very complete indexes, thank heavens. And don't forget one other key option: Ask someone who does similar procedures what they've discovered about shortcuts.

❖ ❖ ❖ ❖

Right away, learn how to use macros that can reduce complicated, repetitious tasks to a single keystroke wherever you can. Programming and editing them is usually easy these days, and the half hour spent setting up a fairly complex procedural or textual macro can save you hours down the road.

Preventing Computer Problems

Keep the computer cool and make sure it has air flow around it (if it's a laptop, *under* it).

❖ ❖ ❖ ❖

Dust your computer every so often. You can vacuum a keyboard, or use an eraser pencil brush on it. Vacuum the vents on the side of the computer, too. When they get clogged with dust, the computer gets too hot.

IF YOU NEED COMPUTER TRAINING

When office workers need computer training, single-shot, intensive training sessions can be a mistake. They can be frightening, overwhelming — just watch people's eyeballs roll back in their heads.

Companies throw buckets of money away when they send five people from the same office to an expensive one-day seminar (where you'll learn a lot you'll never use, and the teacher crams as much as possible in). Instead, ask your company to pay your tuition for a semester-long evening course at a local community college. In return, offer to pass on the important skills to coworkers.

Clean your mouse regularly. There are optical mice available with no moveable parts, so they can't get dirt or hair in them. And Logitec, for one, makes a mouse that is sealed so it can't be fouled with crud.

❖ ❖ ❖ ❖

There are cleaners available for CD and disk drives, and your drives will last longer and give you less problems if you use them.

Make "Save. . . Save. . . Save" your mantra.

Optimize once a week, using a program like Norton Utilities, and your hard drive will rarely fail. Optimizing lines up all the file segments in your computer so it can find them faster.

❖ ❖ ❖ ❖

To make sure all the wires and plugs end up back in the right place when moving a computer: First, make sure the computer is turned completely off, and then take masking tape and put a piece on every wire and occupied port. Put matching identifying numbers on each part.

The safest surge protector for a computer is an uninterrupted power supply (UPS) box. In addition to evening out the power supply, and protecting the computer from power sags and surges, which can cause severe damage, a UPS will power the computer in the case of a power outage. This will give you time to properly close the applications you're using, and to save and prevent loss of data. (However, a UPS won't do you any good if you aren't there to see the power go off.) Not everyone in an office needs a UPS, but if you think you do, make the case to your manager or the company's systems professional.

❖ ❖ ❖ ❖

Most printers use too much power to be plugged into a UPS. They should be plugged into a good-quality surge-suppressor outlet. Many "power strips" are no more than extension cords, and should not be depended on to protect against storm damage.

❖ ❖ ❖ ❖

Don't spend a lot on an expensive surge protector. They all do the same thing and none of them will protect you from a direct lightning strike.

❖ ❖ ❖ ❖

In a thunderstorm, don't just turn the computer off — unplug it. Unplug the phone line to your computer, too, or a lightning zap could travel in on the modem.

Keep your floppy disks or backup tapes safe:

- Don't put them in the sun or near any other source of heat.
- Don't let them get wet. (Coffee can kill.)
- Keep them away from magnets (the surface of a disk or tape accepts magnetic charges, and a magnet changes the configuration, causing the data to be lost or garbled).
- Store backups in another office or building. Fires and other catastrophes happen, and having your backup disks in the bottom drawer of your desk won't help you if your workstation gets seriously damaged.

WHEN SOMETHING GOES HAYWIRE

- If something goes wrong with your computer, write down what you were doing when it happened. Carefully copy down any messages the computer gives you — it will usually try to tell you what's wrong. Even if you can't decipher them, they'll help the person you call to fix the computer.
- Most breakdowns are software generated. To prepare for breakdowns, save and back up. Optimize. Use virus protection. If you figure out a fix, write it down *on paper,* because the same thing may happen again.

Never send a piece of paper through a laser printer twice. Paper in a printer of this type is subjected to intense heat, and when things are heated up they get crispy. On that second trip through, tiny particles will fall off the surface of the paper into the printer and gunk it up, which will eventually cause problems.

❖ ❖ ❖ ❖

If you have an ink-jet printer, be sure to use paper designed for it, or you'll have smearing problems.

❖ ❖ ❖ ❖

Keep a "boot disk" with all of your system start-up software on it so that if your hard drive crashes, you'll be able to start the computer from the disk drive, load new software, or run a diagnostic on it.

Health Maintenance (Yours)

When working at the computer, sit up, and maintain good posture. Raise your monitor up on a box if necessary to help you work without straining. Adjust your chair height and the angle of the monitor screen. If glare bothers you, don't just suffer with it. Adjust the screen brightness and background, change the lighting arrangements, or move the monitor elsewhere.

If you spend a lot of time at a computer, make sure the focal length of your eyeglasses is right for this — it's different from reading distance and general seeing. Otherwise, you may end up with a bad headache.

❖ ❖ ❖ ❖

If you're nearsighted and wear bifocals, consider having a pair made up that's not bifocal, one that puts the keyboard, monitor, and copy stand into perfect focus and lets the distance go hazy. It'll save you all those little jerking head movements as you switch lens zones.

❖ ❖ ❖ ❖

You might want to consider a trackball rather than a mouse, so you can use your thumb instead of your whole hand. Your arm won't be going all over the place, and you won't be using your hands as much and making repetitive motions. Glide pads are good for the same reason.

❖ ❖ ❖ ❖

You can buy all kinds of "wrist rests" and pads to help prevent repetitive stress syndrome, but a towel rolled or folded into a pad of the size and shape you need will do just as well. It'll be more absorbent, too, and you'll be able to wash it!

The Last Word Is You

Remember, you're the Programmer! From a competent person, I heard something that made me flinch. I was in the throcs of making one of those big decisions and he said, "Don't sweat it, the computer will tell you where you're going." But computers are only information processors and tools — they can't weigh values and make judgments. When you start shrugging your "situations" onto a computer, expecting it to tell you what you should do, your productivity, management, and quality of work will eventually skid. Direction is a personal decision, not a question of odds or economics.

6

The Telephone

In this chapter . . .

- *Simple Time-Savers*
- *Clearing the Lines*
- *Voice Mail*
- *Car Phones*

A ge gives us the advantage of living history instead of reading it. I lived way out in the boonies as a child, and we had no phone. In fact, no one in the community did. Then the local schoolhouse got one, the crank type, in the vestibule, and everyone in town used it.

When our family got a phone, it was a seven-party line (great for intrigue, but forget efficiency). Then we got a private phone, a "number, please" format, and finally a dial phone. After that, technology really took over. We got an extension or two, a wall phone, shop phone, then underground cable, Touch-Tone, an answering machine, call-waiting, caller ID, and dozens of long-distance companies plaguing us nonstop for our business.

In the office we now have a $40,000 integrated phone system that we all have to go to classes to learn to operate. The result: The phone has become both a wonder and a powerful distraction.

THE FREQUENT CHATTERS' CLUB

Stop and analyze your last twenty or thirty calls and why you made or took them, what was said and when they came. I think you'll discover that if things had been planned or done sooner, or clearer instructions given, most of these conversations would not have been necessary.

The simple moral: If you join the Frequent Chatters' Club, you will have to pay the dues.

A corollary: You have to pay triple damages if you join the Frequent Cellular Chatters' Club.

Simple Time-Savers

Programming frequently called numbers may save only five or ten seconds on each call, but that adds up to a lot of hours over time. Reduces dialing errors, too.

❖ ❖ ❖ ❖

We've all been accidentally cut off on a business call more times than we'd care to count up, usually because someone forgot to push "hold" or pushed another button instead. So pay attention to what you're pressing, and do say, "Before I switch you, the extension is ___, in case you get cut off."

Take some time to practice and experiment with the system — for example, have a friend call and practice transferring them.

❖ ❖ ❖ ❖

After you've made a little preparatory outline for that important phone conversation (see page 33), write the phone number you'll be calling on top of the page. If you get a busy signal or have to call back later, the number will be handy for the next attempt.

❖ ❖ ❖ ❖

If you have more frequently called numbers than your phone's memory can handle, make a cardboard-mounted, one-page sheet of the extra numbers (add addresses while you're at it).

❖ ❖ ❖ ❖

If you often use a computer and a phone simultaneously, a headset phone is terrific! Even better, try a *portable* headset phone so you can walk around with it on. It frees both hands to write, reach for needed materials, check files, and the like. Saves contortionist cramping of hand, neck, and shoulder.

Phones don't have the right, but they do have the might, to invade our day anytime and anywhere. . . if we let them.

A daily log of significant phone calls noted in a steno pad or kept on computer can be a big help. That way you have a record and can easily go back when someone asks, "When did so-and-so call?"

"BOB CALLED. . ."

It's one of the things we're always cussing ourselves and others about: sloppy message taking!

How often have you been unable to decipher an important message you took yourself or someone gave you? The phone number is wrong or unreadable, you can't remember what those scribbled abbreviations meant, you didn't get the name, or it isn't spelled right. Or the message is just plain too short: "Bob called!" Bob who? I know at least thirty Bobs! And by the way, what did Bob call ABOUT?

It doesn't take a bit of skill, extra brain power, or training to correct this. Take fifteen seconds more on the next message to do it right, and watch how it simplifies things!

Clearing the Lines

One unnecessary tie-up of a work phone is one too many. Some potential customers or clients will only call once as they work their way down the Yellow Pages. Too often an overly lengthy work call or, worse, a personal call can destroy an opportunity. Limiting the length of personal calls on business phones is a significant simplifier.

❖ ❖ ❖ ❖

If we haven't already, we need to train our family and friends not to call us at work except in emergencies.

❖ ❖ ❖ ❖

As for those inside-the-company calls, after a while we get a sense for who is calling to kill time and whose calls are useful. If a call comes in from a time killer, start talking seriously about some company projects or priorities, until the person realizes this is too much like work, I don't want to do this, and gets off.

❖ ❖ ❖ ❖

Many problematic calls that never seem to end may be from people you really want to hear out or about things that really interest you. The problem is the poor timing, not the poor caller. The answer? "I'd love to hear more about that, when I'm not as tightly scheduled as I am today." If this is a business issue, add: "Why don't you write that up and send it to me? I'll get back to you, and we'll get together when I have more time." This puts the situation in your hands, and better yet, it usually brings the caller quickly to the point.

❖ ❖ ❖ ❖

If you're frequently pestered by people asking for your opinion on things within the scope of your profession, tell them you do consulting work on that for a hundred dollars an hour. Or tell them you can answer them much better if they write up the question or the situation with some background and mail it to you. Having to go to the trouble of writing something up will thin the ranks of the inquirers considerably. Calling is easy; writing is work!

❖ ❖ ❖ ❖

We need to have a quick and solid response ready for phone solicitors. Write out a series of standard excuses, if necessary — "Sorry, I'm fully invested," or "Our company policy prohibits accepting free gifts." Immediately add some tiny kind note, such as "Thanks for checking with me, anyway." It's easy to do and removes the sting. Then say goodbye and hang up as fast as possible.

❖ ❖ ❖ ❖

One of the best ways to control calls is to establish a time each day, or certain days of the week, when you receive and return calls. Then make sure your regular contacts know about it. If you have an assistant to screen calls, he or she can help get the word out to familiar callers. Better yet, take advantage of voice mail.

❖ ❖ ❖ ❖

Don't be afraid to forward your calls directly to voice mail during certain key hours. No phone ringing will increase your productivity tremendously.

Rules for Conference Calls

Conference calls work well up to the level of, say, eight or nine people. Beyond that, some people clam up and others come away thinking they couldn't get a word in edgewise. So they call back later for a one-on-one, which defeats the purpose. Here are half a dozen simplifying suggestions:

1. Have an agenda, send it to all participants ahead of time, and stick to it. Brainstorming can make two expensive hours disappear fast.

2. Record the operator's number just in case you get dropped off and can't manage to get back on.

3. Arrange for someone to take notes on the conversation.

4. Be sure to have an assertive facilitator to introduce people, lay out the ground rules, keep things organized, interrupt if necessary, and redirect the conversation.

5. Identify yourself before speaking

6. The more noise people make in the background, such as folding paper, moving chairs, and tapping pens, the harder it will be to hear what is being said.

Above all, if you're not comfortable with conference calls, don't try to finalize commitments or make other binding decisions during them.

Voice Mail

Voice mail came about after studies showed that when you call a company, more than half the time you don't reach the person you want. Far superior to an answering machine, voice mail can do much more than most people use it for. Time spent learning your company's voice mail system can really pay off. Take advantage of these keep-work-simple features by learning how to:

- Leave a complete, clear message. Practice by leaving one to *yourself* (then have a friend, spouse, or colleague critique your etiquette).
- Dictate a quick letter for an assistant to send.
- Forward calls to colleagues' voice mail.
- Retrieve messages from home or the road.

Car Phones

Driving while using a car phone can be a major safety hazard. Emergencies are one thing, but casual conversations and poorly prepared business calls are quite another. Most car phone calls should be made after you've pulled off the road or parked.

❖ ❖ ❖ ❖

In some businesses and circumstances, car phones *can* be a real asset. But having them when we don't really need them means another thing to pay for, hunt for, tend, lock up, and be interrupted by. All in all, making work harder, not simpler.

7

Corresponding

In this chapter . . .

- *E-mail Pointers*
- *Memos, Copies, and Reports*
- *Mailing*

I've noticed that really successful people often write their reply right on the bottom of the letter I sent them. That's fast, easy, compact, complete, *simple* — I love it.

❖ ❖ ❖ ❖

"Hasn't the computer made letter-writing much simpler?" you may be wondering, yet I see many people around the office spend even more time and money on letters since they got their computer with all its accessories. When things get easy, it seems that we always manage to find another way to "overkill." (If, however, you have a good, simple-to-use spell-checker program, *use* it!)

The beginning, middle, and end of simplifying correspondence:

1. Get the message across quickly.
2. Convey some personality and warmth doing it.
3. Get it there fast and cheap.

❖ ❖ ❖ ❖

A quick, very brief letter is better than a long delay while you're waiting for time to write a longer, more thoughtful one. So develop some succinct one or two-liners for when they're needed, such as: "We have your proposal and will try to reply by the end of the month," or "Some of us liked your idea, but others find it too expensive, so we must pass."

❖ ❖ ❖ ❖

Don't write unless you have to. It may be cheaper to make a quick call (even a long-distance one) to give an answer. Or better yet, use E-mail when you can.

❖ ❖ ❖ ❖

If you find yourself writing certain types of letters over and over, create merge form letters, with "stops" at points that need personalizing. Keep all of your form letters in a separate subdirectory. If customized letters are not essential for your business, you may wish to use preprinted form letters.

If you E-mail similar material frequently, use your word-processing software to create your own "Personalized Speed Macro" form.

❖ ❖ ❖ ❖

If it's not possible to get a letter typed or printed, a handwritten note may be not only effective, but even more personal and graceful.

❖ ❖ ❖ ❖

Even with the aid of the swift and tireless computer, correcting things takes time. How many errors justify revising and reprinting a letter you thought was ready to go? One hand-done correction on a piece of correspondence is okay — in fact it adds a personal touch, as well as the assurance that you actually read it before it went out.

❖ ❖ ❖ ❖

Don't apologize at length in a business letter for something minor, such as delay in answering. It wastes time, and just reminds readers of their irritation. They've heard from you at last, and what they're really interested in is the point, which you have not yet gotten to! If you feel apologizing is essential, do it just once, briefly — and remember that one *good* excuse is usually better than two or three.

❖ ❖ ❖ ❖

When registering complaints, brevity beats the blow-by-blow. "We relied on you and it didn't turn out well" is usually better than taking the time and energy to get down all the details, eager as you may be to immortalize every irritating shortcoming.

❖ ❖ ❖ ❖

Thanks to those marvelous computers, we can send formal letters or E-mail to forty-two people in no time flat, just by popping in names and addresses. This operation is so simple it's almost brainless, wherein lies the catch: It's all too easy to ship out the wrong message or materials packet to the wrong person. Always double-check before you post or transmit!

ACRONYMS AND JARGON

When I see an ASAP
What does that symbol mean to me?
Some codes, such as these FYIs,
Seem understood by other guys.
As for FOB, I might decipher this
But AOL-LOL I surely miss.
"ADC pulled a JIT" — what are you really
  telling me?
"ID the V/SOT" is total Greek, you see.
Acronyms and jargon are new and nineties
      — hot!
But more efficient? ITN! (I think not!)

E-Mail Pointers

Bypass the fax, go E-mail whenever possible. You can send E-mail to groups of people simultaneously, such as the executive committee, all district managers, your immediate family or extended family. You can send blind copies or courtesy copies, so that people will know or not know who else got it.

❖ ❖ ❖ ❖

If you find yourself getting swamped with E-mail, there are E-mail programs available that sort types of messages (business, personal, etc.), enabling you to read the most important messages first.

❖ ❖ ❖ ❖

Purchase a program that transfers messages to a laptop, so you can review messages while en route to meetings or on the road.

❖ ❖ ❖ ❖

Read and respond to only the most recent of a group dialog generated in E-mail.

❖ ❖ ❖ ❖

Try to keep a clean slate. Delete E-mails that you have responded to if you don't need to keep a record of them.

❖ ❖ ❖ ❖

If you need to keep an E-mail, don't print it out. That defeats the purpose of time-saving, space-saving electronic files. Instead, create topic folders in your computer files and store E-mail messages in the appropriate files. That way, they're there when you need them and you've saved a tree or two.

❖ ❖ ❖ ❖

Schedule a couple of times a day to concentrate on catching up with your E-mail. If you don't, you'll respond to every little beep that signals "incoming," feel constantly interrupted, and perhaps lose that once-in-a-lifetime thought that you were just about to capture.

❖ ❖ ❖ ❖

If you have a modem, a way of dialing into your office network, and a home computer, you can access your E-mail in the relative peace of your home. Talk to your office systems manager and see if this is available to you. It can be a lifesaver if you work at home occasionally or if you're on the road with a laptop. No more arriving back at the office to find 89 unread E-mail messages!

❖ ❖ ❖ ❖

Set up electronic "user lists" for the members of any committees you might be on. If you have an idea or want to get feedback on a suggestion, or just keep other members up to date, broadcast it to the user list that applies. This is simple, keeps everyone informed, and meetings will take less time and be more productive.

If you are creating an important memo, draft it on your word-processing program rather than creating it directly in E-mail. You can keep it on your computer for further reference. In E-mail, simply attach it to a short message and send it off to the appropriate people. By the way, they can save it in their computer filing system, too, rather than delete it from their message log.

Memos, Copies, and Reports

I read all memos, but I've noticed that some people read few or none. "Why?" I've asked. The answer: "Too many, too often, too long, too inapplicable." They're right. Many of the memos I've faithfully plowed through have been all of the above. Don't ever establish a reputation for memos that just become moss covered. Not only will your memos go unheeded, people will begin to treat you the same way. Keep your memos simple, conversational, and short, and distribute them selectively.

❖ ❖ ❖ ❖

Yes, everyone wants your autograph, even in your own office. Who doesn't receive notes, memos, and requests with missing names or dates? After many years of working together at the office, our style gets ever more casual and informal. I often get requests but haven't a clue who they came from or who to give them back to.

- Don't count on your handwriting style alone to identify you. In our office there are three people who write very much alike.
- Include your last name. We now have two Kathys, three Daves, two Marks, and three Lanas.
- Initials can't be counted on, either. I've created major confusion directing notes to "CC" (is it the Cleaning Center, my store, or my coauthor, Carol Cartaino?).
- Always date things, too. Trying to figure out "when" can be just as confusing as trying to find out "who."
- And include the year. It may seem unnecessary at the time, but years pass quickly, and many inadequately dated items — clippings from newspapers and magazines, for instance — can become enigmas in the file.

❖ ❖ ❖ ❖

Copies of actual transactions can be better than memos! There's an efficiency factor here that too few take advantage of. Copies are cheap, easily routed, faster than memos, and contain dates, names, the action taken, and who did it. Many times, simply distributing copies will let you fill people in completely without your saying a word, making a call, or holding a meeting. Copies are a polite way to create awareness and teamwork, to share compliments and progress, and even to toot your own horn.

❖ ❖ ❖ ❖

The simple secret of a good report: Don't include more information than was asked for, or is needed!

If your cabinetmaker proudly showed you the rough, unfinished box that would eventually become the planed, sanded, and varnished new kitchen cabinet you ordered, you would probably realize that he planned to complete the job, and not be alarmed. But if you, the writer-carpenter, show a rough draft of a report or proposal to others, they may think you aren't a very good writer, or that your presentation leaves a lot to be desired, even if you tell them it's unfinished. So keep the rough stuff to yourself, whenever possible.

STRUNK AND WHITE, CONDENSED

If you don't have time to read William Strunk and E.B. White's *Elements of Style,* which has cured many people of bad writing, here's their message in a nutshell:

- Replace business jargon and stiff "official" phrases with plain English.
- Use one- or two-syllable words, not long fancy ones.
- Write in short, simple sentences.
- Use the active rather than the passive voice.
- Get to the point.

Reports and memos: Remember that making tracks (moving ahead) is better than keeping track. One is active, the other passive. The active is what feeds the passive — activities like chronicling and record keeping. If you don't make any tracks, there won't be anything to keep track of, so keep this first and foremost in your mind. The goal is to make the news, not write or read it.

Mailing

In the computer age we can easily forget that the intelligent, timely use of mail can still greatly simplify office work. Moreover, it's easy to create, 99 percent reliable, private, seldom misunderstood, and cheap. It allows clients and customers the time and dignity to answer, provides a clear record of communications, and, in my experience, generally results in better decisions than faxes and phone calls.

❖ ❖ ❖ ❖

Let the post office help you! Before doing large business mailings (two hundred or more pieces), check out the many (at least sixty-seven!) different discounts the post office has for mailings provided to them in particular ways, such as with the bar codes already on them or presorted in certain ways. Many businesses do not bother to do this, and it can save a lot of money.

❖ ❖ ❖ ❖

The post office has a business center in Phoenix that can provide all the information you need regarding mailing requirements. The number is 1-800-223-3535. If you're designing a mailing piece, just call and explain what you're doing and they'll give you someone who can help. They can provide things like templates that show minimum and maximum sizes for letters and postcards, and correct placement of addresses.

❖ ❖ ❖ ❖

If you find yourself forever sending things by overnight express, priority mail, or Saturday delivery, you might take a look at the underlying reasons. How much of that "speedy sending" is not fully necessary, should never have been necessary, or ends up wasted? There are aging piles of priority and express envelopes lying unopened in more offices than we would want to know about, even as we are carrying our latest offering to the Fed Ex counter.

❖ ❖ ❖ ❖

When does fast really matter? Good reasons for speed:

- Someone desperately needs something to preserve their health or life, or they can't proceed without it — medicine or medical report; part for computer, truck, or tractor; set of spectacles to replace one lost or broken.
- Something perishable has to get there before spoiling.
- A customer or client is really eager for something, willing to pay for speed, and it's worth our while to supply it.

TIPS FROM THE POSTMASTER

Here are some super mail-service simplifiers from a seasoned postmaster:

- Use zip codes. It's surprising how often they are omitted.
- Omit punctuation in addresses and return addresses, and use abbreviations.
- The machines that sort mail today always read bottom to top; don't write below the line with the zip code on it.
- If you send mail to street addresses in towns where only P.O. boxes are used, your mail may get returned to you. (Although in a small town the P.O. might try to deliver them anyway.)
- Don't put things like metal paper clamps, badges or buttons, or loose coins in regular envelopes, which may end up mangled by the sorting machinery.
- Never put Scotch tape over stamps; it voids them since they can't be canceled.
- Arrows all over a package saying "This Side Up" are pointless, as is writing "Fragile," since the package will be thrown into a sack, the sack will be tossed onto a truck, then thrown onto a big conveyor, and so on.

Keeping Things Moving

Henry Ford made more than cars, he made us aware of the advantages of capitalizing on and maximizing "flow" at the workplace. His theory was simple: Things went in one direction, in clearly defined steps and stages that efficiently turned a basic framework into a finished product.

When you think about it, we at any office job "manufacture" an end product, too, and everything should have a clear route toward that objective. Our correspondence, in/out-boxes, filing and storage systems, schedules, and so on, are all part of this pathway, which serves not only to aid and organize us but to keep others informed so that they can help us build that end product. Ford's assembly line moved right along, as we should and can if we have some simple processing systems in place.

There are really no "secrets" for running things flawlessly — probably 95 percent of us already have the knowledge and ability to do this. It's mainly a matter of enacting the things we already know ought to be done, *when* they should be.

Let's take a look at some simple ideas that can aid your quest for a smoother operation.

Three Rs: Reading, Routing, and Remembering

Master the magazine oversupply. Select two or three (mailed or on-line) that really zero in on your career or professional interests, and maybe another general interest one that gives you insights worth having. Forget the ten thousand others, especially the free ones that take your time but provide nothing except advertising in return. Then process each issue — read or scan and rip out anything really valuable (making sure to note the date and issue number on it) — within hours of receiving it. Saving just means stacking when it comes to magazines.

❖ ❖ ❖ ❖

Direct mail isn't all "junk." It can help keep us aware of things we didn't know about. But it has to be controlled. Skim and chuck, unless you have an assistant who can ruthlessly presort it.

It seems logical to work from the top of a reading pile down, whether it's reports on your desk or E-mail that you've let linger, but that pile got there by placement, not priority. So before picking anything off the top, riffle through the whole pile quickly and pull out the item that really needs your attention first.

❖ ❖ ❖ ❖

Clear out the cash! The longer something that belongs somewhere else "sits," the greater the risk it will be lost, forgotten, or damaged. Especially money. When checks, cash, money orders, or credit card charges are received, get them to the bank or wherever else they're supposed to go immediately. Hiding things like this away or storing them up for a deposit is just asking for complications. Make sure that money is where it should be, when it should be. Cash and credit transactions carry a sure sentence of accountability with them — any mistake we make is twice as hard on us as even a major mistake with personnel or reports.

❖ ❖ ❖ ❖

Even the largest and most hidebound organization usually has some procedure for getting out a payment quickly. Find out how to "walk through" a check when you need to — but don't overuse this privilege, or you won't get any cooperation next time.

If you do a lot of routing of things to different branches or outposts of the company, it's usually more efficient to have a pocket, bin, basket, or slot in the wall for things going to these different destinations, so you can collect and batch things, rather than having everyone constantly sending individual pieces.

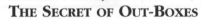

THE SECRET OF OUT-BOXES

You can have a 50 percent simpler in-out system immediately — get rid of the out-box. What good is it? Anything finished or going out shouldn't be sitting in a box. Out should mean under way, on the way to its destination, so get it gone when you get it done.

One of the smartest lists and records we keep is an address book. From black book to laptop directory, having the right address and phone number at our fingertips is one of the best time-savers and simplifiers. If you want to make your own directory, just come up with a format or layout for it, put it on the computer, and print out several copies: one to carry (no one *always* has a laptop handy), one to leave in the office (computers *do* go down), one for home or for your spouse, one for each of your close office staff. On the one you carry, fill only the top three-fourths of the page, leaving the bottom blank for on-the-spot additions. Leave room, too, to alter existing entries. Get any changes into your computer as soon as convenient. Then review the whole directory at least annually.

❖ ❖ ❖ ❖

Answer questions before they get asked. Be careful not to send papers or documents out to people with no explanation. This happens because we're often so familiar with the content that we forget the needs of the reader. So:

- Include a little note explaining what you're sending and/or what the receiver should do with it.
- Note how many copies are enclosed, and how many must be returned. If some part of the enclosure needs to be signed or initialed and/or notarized and returned, make sure you clearly note it. If necessary, explain step by step what you need done.
- If the document includes legal or other terms or phrases that the average person may not understand, give a quick translation.
- Call the receiver's attention to any critical performance deadlines or appearance dates included in the document.

❖ ❖ ❖ ❖

Getting people to sign and initial all the right places is an important part of processing official documents of all kinds, but this seemingly simple matter is anything but simple in practice.

The very best way to make sure all important papers get the proper signatures on them is still to stand over them and make sure it happens. But when that isn't practical (it usually isn't), try putting penciled Xs in all the pertinent spots or using rubber stamps, such as "Initial Here," to direct attention. Or try brightly colored tags, such as those made by Post-it, that stick out prominently from the sides of the paper. Some are even printed with instructions, such as "Please sign and date."

❖ ❖ ❖ ❖

One valuable thing I've learned from having years of multiple projects and assignments poured on me is to take all the key names, numbers, addresses, and objectives of a project and put them on one sheet or a single manila folder or a single computer file page, so I have everything and everyone I need to remember, call, or contact in one spot. It will take you a few minutes to clip and paste or edit it all together, but once you have it all "indexed" like this, you'll save hours of hunting and sorting. And when you want someone to help, it only takes two seconds to hand them the sheet or E-mail the page.

❖ ❖ ❖ ❖

Tickler files for follow-up: Many of us already have these, to keep us aware of commitments and to-dos coming due next week or three months from now. To keep us timely, we need to put those reminders in far enough ahead of the actual due date to give us time to accomplish it comfortably. We can also use ticklers in a more positive, big-picture way, to remind ourselves to carry through on bright ideas that may not come to bear until some far point in the future. Don't hesitate to tickle yourself well into the twenty-first century.

Filing

Filing carries a bad aura, mostly because we're usually behind in it. But think of what filing actually means and can do for us! What a feeling of confidence and security it gives to be able to actually find things. Otherwise, all is out of control.

❖ ❖ ❖ ❖

Files have to be designed so that they are intelligible to everyone. Best to have a brainstorming session before setting up or revising a system so people don't have to be puzzling over some weird set of labels or categories.

❖ ❖ ❖ ❖

When naming files, stop and think a minute before writing your first impulse on the file tab or entering it into the computer. Are you sure you're leading with the true key word?

❖ ❖ ❖ ❖

Don't get caught up in cute or cryptic names for your computer files and subdirectories. And don't count on date alone to remain meaningful. As time passes, the virtues of simple comprehensibility at a glance will become clearer and clearer. Your computer's operating system (Microsoft's DOS, for example) used to limit file names to eight characters and a three-character extension, but a lot of software has overcome that limitation. If your software has, take advantage of it. A file you can identify as "Slothrup Initial Proposal Feb 13 97" beats "initprop.F97" any day.

❖ ❖ ❖ ❖

With files of paperwork I carry around or use often, I don't depend on the those little tabs for identification. I label the outside of the folder in felt tip pen with big, bold letters.

❖ ❖ ❖ ❖

Getting behind just means stacks and piles (or overlooked computer subdirectories) to oppress us! The day we say we're going to "catch up the filing" is usually the day something major suddenly has to be done right away. When it comes to paper, the smartest approach is never to go home at night or start work in the morning until 100 percent of everything worthwhile is filed or refiled. If you can't keep up daily, you need to catch up at least twice a week. You never know when you will need something in the stack. Or two dozen people will be wasting time in a meeting while you try to find it.

❖ ❖ ❖ ❖

Things misfiled or left in the wrong computer directory under a forgotten, illogical name might as well be lost in space. This is largely a result of waiting — piling things up or letting them lay around.

Self-Reliance

The simplest of all work-simplifying secrets: do it yourself. People keep trying to convince us that success and simplicity mean getting someone else to do all the labor while we stand there with a clipboard directing and collecting the money. Not so. *Yourself* is the simplest avenue. Maybe you can win the battle before calling in the cavalry!

CAN WE BEAT THE BUREAUCRACY?

Bureaucracy is a great and much-deserved whipping boy. It sure can take the fun out of anything, or keep us from accomplishing it efficiently. But we all have to deal with it, preferably without wasting additional time and effort in fruitless griping.

The cure? Jump through the hoops, but don't get tangled up in them. If office procedure seems to require you to do dumb things, do them as quickly as you can. When the moment is right or the channel available, offer logical shortcuts (in writing, not orally).

Consult yourself before the shelf. Always tap your own intellect and resources before heading for the reference shelf or the Internet. No matter what is out there, what other tools or resources, or what has been done before, by whom, there has never been a "you" before, so don't be afraid to tap your instincts and intellect.

❖ ❖ ❖ ❖

We've all made plenty of speeches and comments about "what ought to be done around here," and most of them fall on unresponsive ears or are made to people with no authority to do anything about the issue in question.

When written up and *signed,* an idea has much greater impact, especially if it comes in the spirit of constructive thinking. If you see something, no matter how obvious or how small, that you think could be changed or improved, go with your first instinct and propose it. Don't assume someone surely must have thought of it already and decided not to do it. This may not only help save the company time and money, but also avoid your dismay when a newcomer comes along and gets rewarded with a bonus for a suggestion that you thought of six years ago.

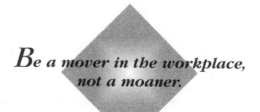

Be a mover in the workplace, not a moaner.

Learn and practice "reserve." Anything you can put a little plus on, do it. Do it even if you aren't paid for it, because it will eventually pay you big dividends. This is the same theory as the old "baker's dozen" — always including a tad over the expectation in case the count falls short. A few examples:

- Money: Always have more with you than you need to get by.
- Make an extra copy to take to the meeting.
- If your manager wants five ideas, come up with seven or eight.
- If you'll be giving a fifteen-minute speech, have an outline for ten minutes more, just in case.
- Keys: One you will lose and one you will leave home, so keep a third backup.
- Human resources: Have handy the name of one more temporary agency, one more freelance keyboarder, one more computer consultant, one more...

SPEAK OUT

Make your path public. Let everyone know your goals, ideas, and plans. Tell people what you are going to do, why, when, how, and where. When people know what you want, they will go out of their way to provide it for you. Silent, secretive people seldom get help, not because they don't deserve it, but because no one knows what they really want or need.

We've all had handled hornets — people who feel they've been dealt an injustice, abused, insulted, or cheated by the company we work for, or one of its products or services. On the phone, in blistering type on the page, or standing in front of you, an angry person is not a simple situation. How do we work it out?

Rule 1. Two angry people is at least four times as bad as just one. Don't let an irate letter or personal confrontation arouse you. Stay kind and cool yourself, and most people will calm down to your temperature if you give them time.

Rule 2. Listen, listen, and then listen some more, in one-on-one privacy, if possible. Take notes, if you wish. Then before you soothe, make offers, or make excuses, ask them, "Is there anything else?" Get it all out before you attempt a repair. It's amazing how the last wave of anger will often answer or heal the first one.

Rule 3. If the facts are on their side, acknowledge the inconvenience, hurt, cost, anguish.

Rule 4. Ask, "What can we do?" Let them suggest the healing course. This will convert them from adversaries to partners in the solution.

Rule 5. Give them a little more than they expect or ask for. If they were shorted a crate of lobster tails, see that they get the crate and a box of stuffed shrimp, too.

Rule 6. Remember, the longer you wait to face the hornets, the bigger the nest!

Your best foresight on a project can be sabotaged by someone else who doesn't do much looking ahead. Remember, it's not all under your own control, and it's wise to allow time for other people to screw up.

❖ ❖ ❖ ❖

Everyone (even the motivation seminar gurus) gets bogged down, bored, or stalemated at times. Flogging away at a project can make anyone want to scream. Scram instead — toss it back in the bin, grab the next item on your project list. The old idea of sticking with things is good, but giving both you and the chore a rest works wonders.

Equipment, Tools, and Supplies

Get and keep the best. We're talking about tools and products here (although the principle also applies to people). Nothing is "a bargain" unless it's a long-term success, not a short-term fix. Yet, "How much is it?" is asked fifty times more often than how well it works and how long it will last. Converting people to "think quality" is a long, hard process — "sale," "reasonably priced," and "available" overrule good judgment at least three-quarters of the time.

❖ ❖ ❖ ❖

Don't buy the line that a newer and fancier tool (especially software!) always makes the job go faster and smoother. Some may, but simple jobs usually don't need sophisticated tools.

DUPLICATE!

The old prospector who had several digs left heavy digging tools and buckets at each site. This saved the labor of packing and carrying. Likewise, we busy people aren't just confined to one office these days. We often work at the branch office, the warehouse, in our car, in the study at home, in bed, at our parents' home, or in the barn.

I do business myself in all these places and have found it wise to keep some key tools (notebook, pencils, tape, letter opener, etc.) at each location. When I have a creative or ambitious moment, I can get right to work rather than run around finding tools. Duplication makes doing easier, and usually it's a tiny investment.

❖ ❖ ❖ ❖

Brand your tools. It isn't the actual cost of a ruler, pair of scissors, cart, or chair that bothers us when someone borrows or loses it, it's simply not having the piece of equipment there when we need it. Our tempers flare, we get disgusted, and we start hunting, asking, and blaming. Things like this can undo us for half a day.

The solution is to brand your tools. Put your name (and your department, too, if necessary) on them in some permanent way. Paint them pink, if you have to! Not for the sheer ego of ownership, but simple convenience. Branding your tools may not be a guarantee against rustlers, but it should help keep things at home on the desk.

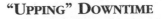

Know how to operate all the office machinery yourself, so you can pitch in and help, if someone doesn't show or you're shorthanded.

"UPPING" DOWNTIME

One of the most important things they teach a new pilot is what to do in a "stall," when the plane suddenly quits flying and sinks like a rock. We do some flying through work, too, and suddenly for some internal or external reason everything shuts down. The job didn't arrive as scheduled, someone doesn't show or call, the flight or meeting is canceled, the electricity goes off, something breaks. We were perfectly prepared and planned, now we've been derailed — downtime.

Pilots in a stall use the speed of the fall to nose into and regain flight at a different altitude. We need to do the same thing. Quickly look at how much downtime you have and pick an appropriate project from your list. Downtime should simply be a fallback and adjustment, not a crash.

Keep an easy-to-read and easy-to-use manual (if it exists!) with every piece of equipment in the office. Concise "how to do it" charts taped to the equipment help, too.

❖ ❖ ❖ ❖

Running out of equipment supplies can have a big ripple effect; it's much more expensive than a little overbuying or overstocking. Making sure we're always ready and able to do our office work is like looking in the cupboard before we start up a recipe — do it up front!

Meetings

Ever notice how it's the unprepared people who use up most of the time in meetings? If you want to simplify and improve meetings, never just go to them. Find out "why" and "what" right after "when." Then take solutions to the meetings, not problems. Written out or sketched-up solutions, not just raw ideas. If you provide a printed summary of your solution, it will be clearer, have more impact, and save everyone from having to take the usual worthless notes. Even if the participants shoot you down, they'll all admire you for the effort, and it will up your "leadership" rating a notch or two.

❖ ❖ ❖ ❖

Hold "Stand-up" meetings. It's a nice opportunity for a stretch, and the meeting will be less likely to take longer than it should.

If a meeting takes more than an hour, you aren't doing it right. Meetings should be well organized, and committee work should be done in committee, not in meetings, which are for presenting summaries and making the important decisions.

❖ ❖ ❖ ❖

If you call a meeting but then realize that a memo would do as well, cancel the meeting and send the memo.

❖ ❖ ❖ ❖

Many view work as a series of social encounters, where it's important to be friendly, supportive, understanding. To avoid conflict, things are not brought to a head. As a result, things remain unresolved, decisions are avoided. Rather than revisiting the same issue a dozen times, get specific. This can be done in hundreds of little ways. Rather than saying, "When you have a chance," say "Could I get that information by noon?" Rather than saying, "Give me whatever kind of report you can," say "How will the information be sorted?" You'll lose few friends, and you'll build respect as someone who knows what they want.

❖ ❖ ❖ ❖

To help a meeting end on time, keep the pressure on, have something scheduled next so it can't run over. Don't let business meetings get too social, which can easily happen if you enjoy the people and the subject.

One of the best kinds of meetings is a business lunch with someone within the company, especially your boss. The more relaxed atmosphere allows a more one-on-one relationship. You can present your arguments full force, without the usual interruptions, and even complain without quite seeming to, in a more conversational way. With a fixed amount of time to fill, the conversation almost inevitably becomes two-way, so you can both develop your concerns or themes at a greater length than you could do in an office setting.

CONFERENCE ROOMS

We're building a new corporate office as we write this book, and a large space in the old building attached to it was tabbed for a conference room. I put out a memo nixing it, explaining how it would serve better as an additional office space, and received back an amazing mass of letters arguing and complaining about not enough "conference room."

My reply included my opinion of conference rooms: "None of us are in business to hold conferences. They are an appendage to production, not production itself. So hold those conferences in your big offices. That will give us shorter meetings and more work done."

9

Dealing with Coworkers

In this chapter . . .

- *The Team Approach*
- *When You Need New Helpers*
- *Office Politics*

I like to exercise my freedoms and feelings at work as well as when I'm off work, just like you. The problem is that everybody, not just you and I, feels that way, and since the office brings us all together, we can easily get in each other's way. When there are seven, seventy, or seven hundred of us on a staff or in a building, reality dictates that we work together as some form of team, with a single purpose and spirit. In this situation unbridled individualism can really muddy the water or ruffle the feathers.

Hence the number one requirement for work efficiency and enjoyment: *compatibility.* Working with coworkers means magnanimity, not just proximity.

The Team Approach

No matter how good we are at our jobs, we often need help around the office, and finding an ally is a smart move toward simplifying work. It can be someone who works with you, for you, or even just around you — someone you can call on when a task is better done by two. Someone who can be trusted to pass on a message in your absence, cover for you, suggest you not send that angry letter, make a joke when you take yourself too seriously.

❖ ❖ ❖ ❖

When you head a team, the ideal assistants are the ones you can give an assignment to and just let them run with it — research things as necessary, and then carry through. To achieve this:

- Make them part of the process of decision making.
- Take them to meetings with you.
- Fill them in on the whole and they'll do their part better.
- Give them specific goals but let *them* tell *you* how they're going to get there.
- Don't do all the interesting work yourself and leave all the boring, brainless stuff for them.
- Give them things that challenge their abilities and knowledge; let them become team experts in some areas.
- Don't let yourself get so busy that you fail to communicate with them regularly (and that doesn't mean once every other week as you're rushing out the door).

If you accomplish a task early, help your team members out. When someone is stuck with a problem, try to help find the solution. Such efforts get reciprocated.

❖ ❖ ❖ ❖

Never make a job indispensable, it's too much pressure for any one person. Arrange things so everyone has relief.

❖ ❖ ❖ ❖

Kind coaxing, or a cuff on the side of the head? The other part of the team hasn't gotten its share of something done, and it's undermining your efforts. The options:

1. Bad: Ask them again and beg and whine for it.
2. Worse: Report them to the boss — you've just made new enemies.
3. Worst: Shame them in front of everyone — you've just made new *eternal* enemies.
4. Marginally better: Do it for them — generally the quickest and simplest solution, but a bad precedent.
5. Best: Diplomacy. Offer to help them do it and schedule time to do so.

❖ ❖ ❖ ❖

Unreliability usually isn't a lack of skill or ability, but of commitment. It can be corrected by nailing down expectations (the job or assignment, its time, the place, the requirements) and then asking just three questions of the person to whom it has been assigned:

- Do you really want to do it?
- Do you have full instructions for it?
- Will you do it?

If the answer to all of the above is yes, wait a while, and ask one question more: *Did* you do it? If the answer is no, you don't need their "help."

GIVING AND GETTING CLEAR INSTRUCTIONS

Let's say you're a willing, ambitious person, arriving fresh and inexperienced on a ranch, and the foreman says simply, "Go get the cows." That's a clear objective but not clear instruction. Whether you're giving instructions or asking for them, strive for clarity:

- Where *are* the cows?
- Do we want them dead or alive?
- Shall I use the pinto or shank's mare?
- What's our brand?
- How many cows are there? What breed?
- Both cows and calves?
- Where should they be corraled? Where do you want them after I get them?

What do we do when the boss is the roadblock? It happens all the time in offices. It's usually better to be honest and businesslike — that is, to exercise diplomacy in its truest sense — than to beat around the bush. If necessary, keep bringing the problem up until it gets addressed.

❖ ❖ ❖ ❖

Sometimes people appreciate praise even more than their paychecks. It doesn't have to be a big thing — just acknowledgment that we are needed is generally enough to fuel camaraderie and cooperation. A thank you is the simplest of all motivators.

❖ ❖ ❖ ❖

Watch for little acts of ingenuity and heroism more zealously than you watch for mistakes. It's amazing how many honest opportunities for praise, public and private, there are out there.

When You Need New Helpers

Two of the most important qualities to look for when hiring personnel:

- The capacity for independent thought (self-reliance!)
- The ability and desire to learn

❖ ❖ ❖ ❖

When there's no room for error, it's better to have an obviously qualified person than someone who "might grow into" the job.

When you have the leeway, consider people not traditionally considered for office jobs. They're often used to working hard and eager to learn.

❖ ❖ ❖ ❖

Many high schools have cooperative business education programs. The students in such programs are available for light office duties part-time a couple of days a week. They are trained in basic business skills, such as word processing, correspondence, and phone handling.

There is also a federal program called Senior Community Service whereby people over fifty-five are available for part-time work for local business. Ask your local senior citizens' council or state employment agency.

❖ ❖ ❖ ❖

Don't let new help become a hindrance! We all get frustrated at times because new people can't yet do things the way we want them done. Often, the assigning, handing off, guiding, evaluating, checking, and rechecking involved in breaking in a helper is more time and trouble than doing it yourself. Instead, start out by working right alongside the helper. You'll be able to evaluate and train *while* the job is getting done.

❖ ❖ ❖ ❖

If you cultivate loyalty you will harvest peace and productivity. Loyalty needs little or no follow-up or pumping up, and won't leave you fed up. Loyalty is a quiet asset too many of us overlook.

Office Politics

The intrigue of a secret link to power, of some hush-hush intelligence floating around the office, is often too juicy to jump away from. It's okay to "tune in to the grapevine," but don't automatically swallow what it produces. And then repeat nothing (though you can ask questions).

❖ ❖ ❖ ❖

If we find ourselves up against office politics, we need to identify which of two kinds we're dealing with. The good kind involves sincere people with different visions of what is best or most profitable for the company. The second kind involves turf wars and the like, and it arises from idleness, boredom, meanness, or sheer competitiveness.

- You can choose to be or not to be a player in the first type, though it's hard to avoid if you've taken on a strong leadership role in your company. If you have no stomach for it, try to stay out of the line of fire.
- The second type is trickier. For instance, others may target you just because they think they look better when coworkers look bad. Don't stoop to their tactics. Maintain your dignity. The truth *does* emerge, but you may need patience.
- Move on if you're working for a place that allows or encourages type two.

There are always three sides to fights and feuds in the workplace:

1. Their side
2. The other side
3. Staying out of it

Always choose number 3, even when friends are involved!

❖ ❖ ❖ ❖

To tone down those interdepartmental wars and office hostilities, avoid "us versus them" attitudes and vocabulary, whether discussing other companies or other departments within your company.

How to tell how welcome you are in someone else's office: Do they offer you a chair?

Try to have no enemies! Some who don't like you will do all they can to complicate your job and make you miserable. If you've needlessly or inadvertently made any enemies, make amends now.

- Don't treat anyone coldly.
- Try not to be sarcastic or short with anyone (we all fall short here).

- Don't deliberately ignore anyone.
- Never give someone the silent treatment (psychologists call this being passive aggressive).
- Speak no ill about anyone to anyone — it *always* gets back!
- Show your appreciation to everyone, and that includes maintenance and janitorial staff, delivery people, vendors, drivers, and security personnel.

❖ ❖ ❖ ❖

If someone at the office says, "Tell this to no one," honor the request, or don't listen. "No one" does not mean one dear and trusted person close to you.

Sexual Harassment and Discrimination

Volumes have been written about sexual harassment and discrimination (racial, religious, ethnic, sexual, and so forth) in the workplace. These are complex, emotional subjects so replete with permutations and complications — ethical, legal, professional, personal — that presenting a brief list of simple rules would risk grossly *over*simplifying them. This book will not do that.

Every company should have in place grievance procedures to deal with allegations of harassment and discrimination. Know what the policies and procedures are, and if necessary, pursue them without delay.

10

Business Travel Far and Near

In this chapter . . .

- *Planning*
- *Travel Arrangements*
- *Your Home Away from Home*

We're as idealistic as can be when sitting in the office laying out a trip, but in reality there's no mercy for mice, men, or managers once we're out in the hands of airplanes, taxis, hotels, restaurants, and conventions.

- Almost nothing runs on time.
- Weather affects both our transportation and our health.
- A day of business travel is at least twice as exhausting as one back at the office.

- You'll have half or a third of the personal time you planned on.
- Any meeting you go to or person you meet with will take twice the allotted time.
- It always costs more than you thought.
- Travel will mean more calls, correspondence, reports, and new solicitations when you get back.

For these and a myriad other reasons, business travel easily ends up more taxing than relaxing. This chapter offers some suggestions to simplify things when you're "on the road again."

Planning

For starters, try these half a dozen quick tips:

1. Set up your schedule as far ahead of time as possible, not days or weeks.
2. If you must take heavy or bulky things with you, ship them ahead early enough to confirm their arrival before you leave.
3. Always take a map.
4. Get emergency numbers.
5. Don't give your contact numbers to everyone. Make inquirers go through someone at the home office to weed out calls that will only distract you or wear you down further.
6. Identify the fastest, cheapest, and easiest way to call in from the road.

When planning how much work to take with you on a business trip, pack all the "for sure" stuff, some "just in case" stuff, and some "behind and catch-up" stuff — for those long nights in the hotel and long hours on the plane.

❖ ❖ ❖ ❖

Forgetting something you need on a trip is bad business. It can do anything from causing you a little discomfort or inconvenience to derailing the whole purpose of your trip. To prevent this, type up and print out a personalized checklist of things you like and need to have with you when you travel. Include both business and personal necessities and niceties, and you might even want to list the key things you need to do to batten the hatches at home before leaving. Then each time you travel you can just run your eye over your "trip list" as you pack, instead of mentally reconstructing the whole assemblage every time.

Keep a duplicate set of toiletries and clothing basics packed and ready to go. Choose clothing that's color coordinated so that you can mix and match and take less. Travel light!

❖ ❖ ❖ ❖

Before traveling abroad, get the address of the American embassy or consulate, and have contingency plans for getting funds in a hurry, covering the cost of medical emergencies, replacing a lost passport, and so on.

Travel Arrangements

If you and other members of your department travel a lot, draw up a checklist for travel arrangements, to make sure no important details get forgotten. The form should address all the pertinent questions, such as flight numbers and times, hotel and car rental reservation, address, emergency numbers, and phone numbers, telephone and fax numbers at your destination, names and phone numbers of contact people, and so forth. Make sure all the blanks on this form are filled in before anyone steps out the door.

❖ ❖ ❖ ❖

Use only one travel agent, and one person at that agency. After a while, that agent will know what you prefer (earliest flight out, window seat, hotel with late-hour room service), and you won't have to go through it all every time.

❖ ❖ ❖ ❖

When making airline reservations, make sure you'll have at least forty-five minutes or an hour between connecting flights. If it's less than thirty minutes, you may be able to sprint the length of 102 gates in some huge airport to make the connection, but your baggage may not have time to be transferred. Everything business travelers carry is important to them, and if you have essential items in those bags, such as props you need for a presentation, you'll be in trouble indeed.

For the same reason, pack whatever presentation materials you can in your carry-on bag. Then, you'll know you have them with you.

❖ ❖ ❖ ❖

Fly with a well-known, well-capitalized airline.

❖ ❖ ❖ ❖

Don't take the last flight into somewhere, if you have any choice at all. If something goes wrong, there will still be at least one more flight to get you and your luggage to your destination that day.

❖ ❖ ❖ ❖

Whenever possible, avoid flights that take you through airports that have a comparatively high risk of closing for bad weather, such as Denver in winter.

❖ ❖ ❖ ❖

Window seats are good, and not just for catching up on cloud-watching. People won't be climbing over you to get in and out of their seats.

❖ ❖ ❖ ❖

Do be sure to check in at the airport an hour before the flight, to avoid being bumped by overbooking. Also, as we know, there's the ever-present threat of construction on the way to the airport, other road delays, those slow-moving shuttles from the parking lot, and big lines at the check-in counter. To avoid this kind of stress, be early, and then you can use that nice serene hour after you're safely there to make phone calls, people-watch, read, write, or nap.

Be nice at the airport, even when things go wrong. Airport and airlines people go far out of their way to assist a nice person. Don't fail to send them thank-you letters when they deserve it. They really appreciate this because they mainly get complaints.

❖ ❖ ❖ ❖

Skip the coffee if you're on a very tight schedule or running late. The extra few minutes it takes for a pit stop could be the ones that make you miss the plane.

❖ ❖ ❖ ❖

Don't wear white or other light colors on route, especially if you're taking any form of public transportation.

Your Home Away from Home

The best place to stay — the most convenient, most efficient, and least stressful — is the hotel that's hosting your convention, meeting, or gathering.

❖ ❖ ❖ ❖

When making a reservation, get not only the name of the hotel or motel chain but the precise name (for example, Holiday North Coliseum, not just Holiday Inn), so everyone including the cab driver will know which of the fourteen Holiday Inns in Dallas is your destination. And since business travelers today don't just stay somewhere but get letters, express packages, and faxes there, make sure you have the full street address and fax number as well as the phone number.

❖ ❖ ❖ ❖

Make sure the hotel spells your name right on the reservation. Otherwise, even if you're able to claim your room when you get there, others may not be able to reach you.

❖ ❖ ❖ ❖

If you're shipping heavy or bulky things, such as presentation props or a big box of training manuals, to someone at a hotel, it can take a little doing to make sure the package isn't lost in space or in the shuffle. Make sure the package is vividly identified in some way, and keep in touch with the hotel's shipping and receiving department so you can find out when the package arrives.

❖ ❖ ❖ ❖

Use room service. It may cost a little more but will save you an hour and a half a day — the time it takes to get presentable enough to go down to the dining room, and the long, boring wait for service at a single table when you get there.

FREE TIME

According to the time experts, travel, including our daily travel to work, takes up two or three years of our lives. I do a lot of business across the continent and across the ocean, and my 1996 average put me on the high end of such statistics, with over seven full days of travel a month. That's eighty-four days (almost three months a year) of just "riding."

When you're away, being transported by air or in a hotel, you're free from "contact" and all those mundane everyday responsibilities of both the office and the home. Once you realize this, leave the food, TV knobs, videos, idle socializing, newspapers, and other trifles alone and hit that to-do list.

If you have a laptop, be sure to take it along. Not only is it great for note taking and other catch-up writing, but you can complete your trip report before you even get home.

11

The Home Office

In this chapter . . .

- *Establishing a Professional Environment*
- *Office Hours*
- *Equipment and Tools*
- *Money Matters*

In the past, "office" smacked of "executive," "official," "professional," "financial." Today, we all have some connection with an office, whether it's in an office building, a garage, or a shop.

Many of us have full-scale home offices having and doing everything that we do downtown, and many folks are running profitable businesses out of the home.

Working at home offers privacy and instant gratification — if you want a snack, a shower, or a nap, you can have it. But most important of all, in your home office you can use the schedule and working methods that are natural to you.

Establishing a Professional Environment

Whether we admit it or not, those of us who have our offices at home sometimes find it hard to feel fully professional. We have no audience to play our official role for: no one around to discuss work problems with, admire our efficiency and ingenuity, and help set a professional tone. Keeping your work space neat and clutter free helps, as does paying some attention to what you look like while you're working. Informal clothes of obvious quality offer a good compromise between the office "uniform" and a bathrobe. (People do sometimes drop in, even at the home office.)

❖ ❖ ❖ ❖

Having a home office intensifies the problem of interruptions, one of the biggest reasons being that people fail to recognize that you're *working*. So they don't hesitate to stop by, hang around, or call. Don't you have time for a chat, a beer, or a cup of coffee? Your very own family, who should be the ones that really understand, are often no better. It doesn't matter what you may be in the middle of, if they need clean jeans for tomorrow or a glass of iced tea now. One solution is to do whatever you can to take the home office *away* from your home. Here are some suggestions:

- Put up a professional-looking sign with your company name on it in a prominent place, such as the door to your office. No hand lettering here please, unless you're a commercial artist or calligrapher.

- Remove as much personal stuff as possible from your office space. This will help assure that it looks businesslike.

- Don't make your office setting *too* warm and friendly — slightly austere and professional is good.

- Put up a bulletin board or marker board in a very visible place and post work-related notices on it, such as, "Deadline March 19th."

- Make sure your business machines, such as the computer and fax, occupy a very visible spot, preferably where they're the first thing people see when they approach the area. Done right, this can have a mildly intimidating effect.

- Make people very aware of when you regularly work. It may take some doing, but they may finally accept that you're "at the office" during those hours.

- When people come or call during your work hours, greet them in a friendly but crisp and businesslike way.

❖ ❖ ❖ ❖

If at all possible (it doesn't really cost that much), have two phones, one for business and the other for personal calls. Answer the business line with the name of your business, and put an answering machine on the other during working hours. Try not to give the business number out to friends and family, not even your mother.

Have both a phone and a fax, and make sure your answering machine message includes instructions for sending faxes. This has an ultrabusinesslike effect.

❖ ❖ ❖ ❖

Avoid the following on your answering machine: musical introductions, a message delivered by a child (no matter how beloved or precocious), very long messages (long-distance callers won't like these), and very clever or cutesy ones. Even the best of these lose their charm, and the listener's patience, after the first or second time.

❖ ❖ ❖ ❖

Decorate your office space with framed or mounted souvenirs of your business successes.

❖ ❖ ❖ ❖

One thing your business callers will really appreciate is a parking place for guests. Many home offices overlook this, which means frustrated clients trying to find somewhere to park, or parking somewhere we wish they hadn't, and neighbors complaining about blocked driveways.

Office Hours

Everyone thinks working at home is the ideal, because you make your own hours, but you may find it the hardest thing you've ever done. Here you must grapple with self-discipline, which is even tougher than trying to please the harshest office taskmaster. There are two basic approaches to scheduling your office time, one of which should suit you:

1. Set a rigid schedule and stick to it no matter what. If there's a TV show you want to see during your working hours, let the VCR do what it was invented to do, and watch the show later.
2. Be flexible, because you can be flexible. Expect interruptions, don't be upset or undone by them. Stop when you really must to soothe a child or fix dinner.

❖ ❖ ❖ ❖

If you find your starting time slipping later and later, the reason can often be traced to availability. The home office usually shares an environment that includes many potential distractions — children, other adults, a kitchen that needs to be cleaned, a lawn, a garden, pets that need care. To minimize these, try the following:

- Work in an area well sealed off from the rest of the mundane reality of home.
- Allot a specific amount of time each day to deal with household distractions and don't deviate from what you decide.
- Make sure everything you need for your job is right there with you, so you rarely have to leave your office. (This may eventually mean having your own bathroom, too.)

If you intend to work seven hours a day, set a working schedule of eight, and assume that one hour of the time will go to interruptions.

THE CHILD FACTOR

We're usually more relaxed, and accomplish more, when we have the satisfaction of knowing our children are happy while we're working. Having your children cared for in your home while you work means luxuries like eating lunch together, taking breaks to check on them, and being nearby in case of emergency. But it also inevitably means more interruptions, so plan your schedule with that in mind.

There are those who say they can work with their children beside them, and this would be great, if truly possible. You might, for example, have a well-stocked play area set up nearby, where the kids could do their thing while you do yours. Or they could play at your feet or, if they're older, even work *with* you on a project. It's worth trying, though perhaps a bit optimistic.

If the work you do would really suffer from having your attention wrested away all too often, you and your children all might be better off if you join the millions of office workers who drop their children at a nanny's, a nursery school, or a day care center in the morning.

We can get so bored being cooped up in our office that we're secretly happy when we run out of toner, because now we have to go to town to get some. But count on one to three hours of lost time every time you do this — time lost to traffic, lines, ogling more office stuff you probably don't need or have room for anyway. All to pick up an insignificant item or two.

❖ ❖ ❖ ❖

Don't use the freedom of the home office to create a prison. Because we set our own schedule, we can take full advantage of the off times, such as weekends and holidays, when the rest of the world is off duty or at play. That means fewer calls and less pressure from the outside world, so we can fire up all cylinders in the peace and quiet and really roll. But don't let this lead you into an endless, unbroken horizon of work, no matter how pressed you are or busy your business may be. Always make time for yourself — there should be a few days in the month for rest, change, and recreation.

Equipment and Tools

The cornerstone of an efficient home office is adequate wiring and power surge protection, to serve and protect that valuable office equipment. We shouldn't be forever struggling to find places to plug in new equipment or having fuses always blowing or circuit breakers tripping. Get a competent electrician to update and upgrade the wiring in your home office, and make sure it includes pro-vision for future equipment with even greater power demands.

❖ ❖ ❖ ❖

The telephone system should also be evaluated, and upgraded to handle multiple lines for phone, fax, modem, and other equipment. (A modem is especially important if you live in a remote location.)

❖ ❖ ❖ ❖

Consider ways to reduce static electricity, such as static-controlling carpeting. Static can seriously affect your equipment's operation.

❖ ❖ ❖ ❖

Answering machines are inexpensive, so have separate ones for personal and business phone lines. You might also consider such service options as call waiting, call forwarding, and caller ID, to dis-tinguish important from annoying calls.

❖ ❖ ❖ ❖

Keep a reserve of key office supplies: an extra car-tridge of toner for the printer and copier, several reams of paper and copy paper, enough checks, maybe even an extra mouse. Running out can cost you time, money, and concentration. And as we've all learned, the nearby small store is usually the most expensive.

When buying computer components and software, consider who will fix it or replace it if something goes wrong, and how dependable the company is. Ask if the seller has toll-free support. If you're spending hundreds or thousands of dollars there, you deserve good service.

BUYING A COMPUTER

If you need to buy a computer, think speed and memory. This means the fastest processor, largest hard drive (certainly no less than a gigabyte), and greatest RAM capacity (no less than sixteen megabytes to start) you can afford. Other essential components include a CD-ROM drive — in the near future most software will be available primarily on CD — and the fastest built-in fax modem available in your selected computer model.

If this seems like overkill, remember that a medium-range computer purchased a few years ago, having, say a 386/25 MHz Intel processor with an 80-megabyte hard drive and 4 megabytes of RAM can't handle even the latest version of Microsoft Windows and an up-to-date word-processing package.

The simple moral: Whatever you buy today will be obsolete long before it wears out.

A corollary: Whatever you buy today will always be cheaper tomorrow.

Don't overspend for a printer or find yourself paying for a brand name. The most important feature of an office printer is the resolution, which should be no less than 600 dpi. Speed, which is a major consideration in a large office where the printer is shared, may not be quite as important in a home office unless you process a large volume of text.

❖ ❖ ❖ ❖

You don't always have to buy new toner cartridges. Some can be refilled at least half a dozen times, at about half the price of new ones.

❖ ❖ ❖ ❖

The world of computers and office technology in general is moving so fast, growing by such leaps and bounds, that everyone who has a home office should try to budget at least a thousand dollars a year just for upgrading software and equipment.

❖ ❖ ❖ ❖

A good, comfortable office chair is absolutely essential. You spend a lot of time in that chair, and it can affect your health as well as your frame of mind. Don't settle for whatever you have available — some thirdhand office reject with broken casters and a spring sticking out of the seat, or a recycled dining room chair. Your chair, in this kind of work, is just as important as your computer!

You don't have to buy office furniture new, at steep prices. In the big town or city near you, there is sure to be a secondhand office furniture store, or more than one. In its huge rooms or several cavernous stories you will find a truly thrilling assemblage of desks, chairs, tables, stands, and credenzas, of all sizes, shapes, styles, and colors. You can outfit your office handsomely for a modest amount. The pieces may not all match, and there may be a chip or scratch here and there, but they'll be sturdier and better made and have more character than most of what you'll see in the latest office catalog.

❖ ❖ ❖ ❖

Don't skimp on lighting. This is especially important if your office is in a dark corner, a basement, or a garage, or if you work a lot at night. Indirect lighting supplemented by task lighting works the best. Fluorescent light is inferior because it fluctuates at high frequency, and can give some people a headache. If you want fluorescents, consider full-spectrum bulbs. They're more expensive, but warmer and more cheerful. Be careful with halogen lights — they get hot enough to burn things.

❖ ❖ ❖ ❖

Set up a simple office mailing station, with all all mailing and packaging supplies together in one place.

❖ ❖ ❖ ❖

To save time and help build a professional image, have rubber stamps made with your company name and address, and other frequently used addresses. For a small charge, your bank will provide you with a "For Deposit Only" stamp that eliminates the need for endorsement.

❖ ❖ ❖ ❖

Whenever the kids see all those neat tools and supplies in your office — your stapler, ruler, calculator, poster board — they instantly want to try them out. And being loving parents, you'll want to indulge them. Don't do it! Equipment ends up broken, misplaced, or lost that way. Instead, buy them their own.

❖ ❖ ❖ ❖

Since clocks don't cost much and we look at them often, pick a clock for your office with a face you like. Don't use a tag-sale clinker with a scratched crystal or one that reminds you of the stern old clock in grade school that never moved. Get one that makes you feel sharp, ambitious, and current. In the home office, especially, psychology is all!

Money Matters

The simplest, most succinct money tip we can offer anyone with a home office, especially if you run your own small business from it, is the following: There are two types of tax systems in the United States — one for the informed and one for the uninformed. Stay informed, and get a dependable accountant and an equally dependable financial planner.

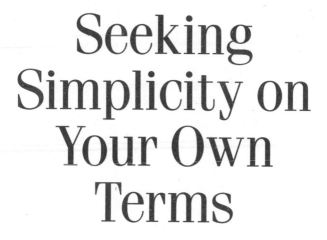

12

Seeking Simplicity on Your Own Terms

In this chapter . . .

- *Preparing to Work*
- *Handling Pressure*
- *Getting Ahead*
- *Defining Success*

A major magazine recently tapped a large group of Americans in their early thirties for a survey. These husbands and wives had one to three children — they were solid, successful families, homeowners with good jobs, respected members of their communities, with plenty of friends and with good health. They were asked just one question: "How are things going?"

The magazine got an answer it didn't expect. Sixty-five percent of those responding were dissatisfied with their job, who they were with, or both. When the respondents were asked why, the consensus was, we did something wrong; we career-planned, but didn't life-plan!

A person with a pulse can get or do almost any job they want, it is loving the job you choose or get that is essential. Life-planning means more than just planning a career with a goal of getting something or somewhere. It means planning to fit who we really are and what we care most about into what we do for a living. This is vital in simplifying work, and if we do it, overcoming the inevitable complications of work will be a challenge, not a chore. If we focus on career alone, we'll force ourselves to perform in a "have to" instead of a "want to" mode, resulting not only in dissatisfaction, but eventually burnout.

Thus the focus of this final chapter is the process of "seeking," not "acquiring." It addresses relatively minor matters, such as how we choose to dress, as well as major concerns, such as defining for ourselves what success means, and seeing to our own mental and physical health along the way. These are all matters that contribute to our self-image as much as or more than our public image. And if we don't pay attention to our welfare on the job, who will?

❖ ❖ ❖ ❖

Sharpen the axe. Some people seem to consistently get more done in less time than others. Are they smarter, or are they chopping with a sharper axe? Schedule breaks in the action... for a moment, an hour, a day, or a week . . . to pause, take stock, and hone the blade. You'll be amazed at how much easier the work goes on your return.

Preparing to Work

What we want in a work wardrobe is apparel that's comfortable for both us and others. Even if you have a dress code where you work, you can choose clothes that make you look good yet are easy to move and sit in. Wear clothes that put you in the mood to roll up your sleeves and work, not stroll down the hall to make sure everyone notices.

❖ ❖ ❖ ❖

Clock yourself to discover your own personal "launching time" — what it takes you to wake up, bathe, dress, get your family ready for the day, take care of other routine responsibilities, and get out of the house. And bear it in mind when making schedules for yourself, especially tightly plotted ones.

❖ ❖ ❖ ❖

Prepare yourself for work the night before, not the morning at hand. Joy in the morning requires some discipline the evening before. This means things like not getting home so late you're bound to be exhausted when the alarm rings. It doesn't end with picking and laying your clothes out, either. It includes reflecting on and mentally readying yourself for the project, the trip, the meeting, the interview. Smart people simplify by preparing and pampering themselves ahead.

To help prevent that sluggish feeling (which can really make office work torture at times), eat the right kind of breakfast and lunch on office days. This means avoiding heavy, rich, fatty food, and foods and beverages with lot of salt, sugar, and caffeine. Alcohol won't do anything for your ambition or alertness, either. Concentrate on fresh fruit, lightly cooked vegetables, salads, low-fat milk products, and moderate servings of fiber-rich whole grain breads and cereals. Don't douse these things with sugar, butter, lots of salad dressing, or jelly, or you're back where you started. And as you're always hearing somewhere, don't skip breakfast!

❖ ❖ ❖ ❖

Some replacements for coffee, when your lids droop:

- Get up to stretch or do a bit of physical exercise.
- Switch to a different chore, or a more energizing part of your current one.
- Munch on raw carrots or celery, apples, sugar-free gum, or big, hard, salt-free pretzels.
- Make a cup of mint tea.

❖ ❖ ❖ ❖

You have to be fit to fiddle! It's become a cliché, but it's still true: exercising regularly tones much more than muscles, heart, and lungs.

When Your Child Gets Sick

For a working parent, the only thing worse than being ill when you have mountains to move at the office is having a sick child. Anyone who has children needs a contingency plan, when staying home simply isn't an option, even though that's what we'd prefer.

- Can you and your mate rearrange work hours to split time at home?

- A grandmother, other near and dear relative, or a friend is the number one resource.

- You can try to do your work from home, but this has its drawbacks. Junior, who has been lying peacefully on the couch all morning, may become clingy and demanding just when that important call is forwarded. If you decide on this plan, be sure to bring home everything you need for the work at hand, concentrate on the tasks only *you* can do, and be prepared to get less done than you imagined.

- If you're lucky, a hospital near you may have a "Kids Sick Room" program. For a low cost you can check your child in here for the day. He'll have nursing attention and be in a cheerful setting that includes TV, video games, all kinds of toys, and even a phone, so that you can check in. Most of the children who have been in a program like this love it, and it has the side benefit of showing them that a hospital is not a place to fear.

If you're the sole occupant of a home office, you might want to work some while under the weather, so everything doesn't pile up on you. But if you work in an office full of people, do your coworkers a favor and stay home if you have a raging cold or the flu — don't bring your germs in and pass them on to everyone else. In *any* office, if you're seriously ill, better to concentrate on getting well than to totter around trying to accomplish something. You'll get well faster, and be back at your post sooner.

Handling Pressure

Stress is not a rare office condition — it infects and endangers millions of us who do office work. But it often has little, really, to do with the work or workload or other people we see as "putting on the pressure." Everyone experiences "pressure," if you want to call it that. Its nicer names are obligation and responsibility, both necessary parts of the pattern of productivity. Doctors, pilots, generals, bus drivers, and parents have a stepped-up version of this "pressure," in that lives depend on their performance, whereas we in an office may only have a deadline or budget to answer to.

❖ ❖ ❖ ❖

If you tend to whine about pressure (tension! strain!), change it. You're the only one who can. You're the one feeling it, you own it, and you can change it by making your job simpler, more efficient, or even by getting a new job.

We seldom feel pressure doing jobs we truly love. The more that is loaded on, or the deeper in we get, the more of a challenge we find it, a victory, even. In reasonable amounts, pressure is a wonderful motivator and disciplinarian. We don't stress out when engaged in worthy endeavors; we get tired, weary, and worn, but we look back at it as "a great time" in our lives. So if we feel a little pressure, we're lucky — it means people value us enough to need us, to expect things from us.

❖ ❖ ❖ ❖

Stress, on the other hand is lots of pressure without any solution in sight. Few will "stress out" if they see or know things will end up okay or be over soon.

❖ ❖ ❖ ❖

If you're sure your stress is malignant, you'd better reexamine why you're at work. If you don't have a few solid reasons beyond a paycheck, you may never be able to simplify your work situation enough to make your life situation endurable.

❖ ❖ ❖ ❖

We can't depend on every manager to create a manageable job; some jobs seem almost designed not to be doable. If you find yourself in this predicament, the best options are to begin looking for another job or to confront your supervisor. If the company wants you to work extraordinarily long hours, ask for additional pay.

If you decide to buy into a heavy-pressure job, you need to do it consciously. How long are you going to do it, at what cost? And for what reason? If your children are now two and four, how old do you want them to be before you have time for them? Are you working to make a million or a name for yourself, or to make yourself and your family comfortable, and enjoy life?

Getting Ahead

Get ahead" is the rallying cry (silent and open) of the office. But many people haven't a clue what "ahead" means in the work environment. Too often, more pay and a higher perch don't turn out to be what we dreamed. Raises, privileges, choices, bigger challenges, flexibility, and freedom are the "ahead" words for me in the world of work. To achieve these there is a simple formula:

1. Do more.
2. Do it better.
3. Earn respect.

❖ ❖ ❖ ❖

There's a lot to be said for stopping your career climb at your level of greatest competence, rather than keeping going until you fulfill the Peter Principle — that people rise to the level at which they become incompetent. You'll be less embarrassed, and happier, too.

Preparing for E Day

I'm amazed how few people know where they stand on their jobs. The incorrect assumption is that it's the supervisor's job to call them in at precisely scheduled intervals and give a readout of how they rate.

No wonder we dread evaluation day at work, when we go into an office or meeting and have our worth summarized on some appraisal form. Pretty brutal if we have no idea what it will say. Dreading the outcome of E day can take the fun out of half a year of work.

You can simplify this situation. That evaluation, after all, is only a report card. It isn't in our manager's hands, but entirely in ours. It's our performance that writes the results. So:

- Have many little E days throughout the year, "expect" days. Frequently ask your manager or supervisor, "Is this what you expect? Am I doing this the way you had in mind?"
- Make sure that you're doing good work, that there are records to show it, and that those records get to whomever does the evaluating.

Then instead of dreading and fearing it, you can show up on E Day for praise and promotion.

Even the Scriptures say, "Let your good works be known." If we don't claim our accomplishments, someone else will. And laying claim after you've been robbed of the credit makes you look like a sorehead. Don't wait to be asked — record your accomplishments.

❖ ❖ ❖ ❖

Never pass up the chance to learn. Our biggest hindrance today is often what we already know: things as they were in the past, that may or may not have any application now. With technology moving so fast, never pass up the chance to learn, even if the subject doesn't seem to be all that relevant to your job right now.

❖ ❖ ❖ ❖

After employing over a hundred thousand people, and teaching several hundred thousand more in seminars and workshops, I've arrived at a simple "Three Needs" to get ahead on the job:

1. *Skill.* Know how to do the job.
2. *Speed.* If you aren't quick and competitive, you'll be culled out or never achieve much.
3. *Tact.* The ability to keep people happy is often overlooked. If you irritate people, you can't work well enough to please them.

EXTRA HOURS

Are extra hours wise? Observation answers that the majority of people who get more done, who make more money, and who are the most trusted and happiest, are the "extra work" type. They are willing, without growling and groaning, to spend a few extra hours when conditions call for it.

Coming in early, staying late, or working an occasional Saturday is about as sensible as it is satisfying. Our workload doesn't watch a clock or obey one, nor are we always able to predict a project's size or length by its due date. And sometimes the office conditions have us *at* the job but not *on* the job, and we need to work early or late or even at home to get our work done.

Extra time at the office offers that real rarity these days, privacy. It always simplifies things when we can move from start to finish with no cutoffs or interruptions. If you're on a roll at 5 P.M., when others are stampeding to the parking lot, it's smart to stick with it an hour or two more, instead of having to spread everything out again and regroup for half a day tomorrow.

Don't be afraid to work some before or after hours — sometimes a well-placed hour can replace a whole day!

Defining Success

Sooner or later we come up against it, the problem of being too valuable to do the fun things anymore. Now that we're worth many dollars an hour, we're too high powered to be wasted researching something to its roots, finding out first-hand what the public out there really has to say, or writing an article for the company newspaper. Or going on business errands where we don't do anything all that important but get to visit interesting places and meet interesting people. This is the price we sometimes pay for getting "up there." But it doesn't have to be so:

- You can find the level you really like best and decide to stay there, "demote" yourself a bit, so you can have projects and not just administration. In other words, carve a niche for yourself that is secure and interesting yet clearly profitable for all. This takes some daring and creativity because the system is geared to the assumption that everyone wants a steady path upward. But if you look carefully, you'll find others already "downscaling" happily, and reaping a reward of respect and satisfaction.

- Decide to do only very highly paid work (even if it's less than fully exciting). Then work intensively enough, long enough, to achieve financial stability, and take lots of time off to do what you *really* want to do.

- Go freelance and only accept jobs you want, so you can enjoy yourself even when working hard. In an era where computerization and downsizing are the hallmarks, this has become increasingly possible.
- Find a way to make enough money to retire altogether while you're still young, and have fun all the time. (Okay, we know this option has never been and never will be realistic for 99.9 percent of us.)
- Realize that the level you're at now is only an intermediate stage, one that you can transcend by systematically moving toward the realms of R&D and entrepreneurship — back to adventure and play!

❖ ❖ ❖ ❖

If all of the above seems a bit ambitious, here's something you can do in the here and now. Take a vacation day and come in to the office anyway — since you're on vacation you should be able to do anything you like. Just make sure everyone *knows* you're "not officially here."

❖ ❖ ❖ ❖

In these pages you may have come to the conclusion that I expect a lot out of people. That's because I know that even the most common persons can do uncommon things if they get through all the politics and protocol, all the "twinking" and thrashing around the periphery of accomplishment. You can do it, and do it today. All it takes is *Keeping Work Simple.*

Index

Other Storey Titles You Will Enjoy

Keeping Life Simple: 7 Guiding Principles, 500 Tips & Ideas, by Karen Levine. Helps the reader assess what's really satisfying and then offers hundreds of pertinent ideas about how to create a lifestyle that is more rewarding and less complicated. 160 pages. Paperback. $9.95 US/$13.95 CAN. ISBN: 0-88266-943-5.

Too Busy to Exercise, by Porter Shimer. Written in a friendly, personal style that both informs and inspires, this book is filled with reasons and ways to fit exercise into the reader's life — regardless of time, space, setting, or equipment. Includes information about nutrition, time-management, and much more. 160 pages. Paperback. $12.95 US/$18.50 CAN. ISBN: 0-88266-936-2.

Too Busy to Clean?, by Patti Barrett. An ingenious collection of simple, clever ways to make cleaning more tolerable and efficient. 128 pages. $9.95 US/$13.95 CAN. ISBN: 0-88266-598-7.

The Rummager's Handbook: Finding, Buying, Cleaning, Fixing, Using, and Selling Secondhand Treasures, by R.S. McClurg. This handbook for a fun and potentially profitable pastime includes hundreds of tips and advice on finding sales, understanding prices, determining value, bargaining, and taking it home. 160 pages. $12.95 US/$18.50 CAN. ISBN: 0-88266-894-3.

These books and other Storey books are available at your bookstore, farm store, garden center, or directly from Storey Publishing, Schoolhouse Road, Pownal, Vermont 05261, or by calling 1-800-441-5700.